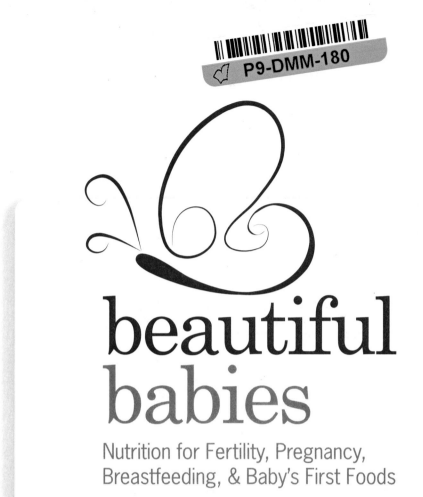

beautiful
babies

Nutrition for Fertility, Pregnancy,
Breastfeeding, & Baby's First Foods

By Kristen Michaelis

Victory Belt Publishing Inc.
Las Vegas

First Published in 2013 by Victory Belt Publishing Inc.

ISBN 13: 978-1-936608-65-2

The information included in this book is for educational purposes only. It is not intended nor implied to be a substitute for professional medical advice. The reader should always consult his or her healthcare provider to determine the appropriateness of the information for their own situation or if they have any questions regarding a medical condition or treatment plan. Reading the information in this book does not create a physician-patient relationship.

Victory Belt ® is a registered trademark of Victory Belt Publishing Inc.

Printed in the USA
RRD 02-13

table of contents

Part One: Nutrition for Fertility, Pregnancy, Breastfeeding, & Baby's First Foods

Part Two: Recipes for Sacred Foods

"Before civilization, humans once had an innate intelligence about what was edible in their environment and how to prepare it in order to extract the most nutrition from it. Kristen Michaelis walks you through the minefield of conventional nutrition babble to the safety of what thousands of years of cultural traditions have shown: that vibrant health comes from eating what our ancestors ate—unprocessed foods from animals raised as they are supposed to live. This is correct nutrition that needs to be taught in every household and school and handed down from parents to children. This book should be required reading for all parents and those contemplating parenthood."

—Jill Tieman MA, DC, CCN, DACBN,
   editor of www.realfoodforager.com

"I want to thank you a hundred times over for the 'Beautiful Babies' e-course. I followed the recommendations that you made and I had a healthy, complication-free pregnancy and birth. I didn't get any stretch marks, varicose veins, no swelling, no pre-eclampsia, etc. I had a water birth with no complications, and I didn't use any painkillers or any drugs! I left the 'birthing center' the same day. I couldn't be happier! Just 1.5 weeks after giving birth and I can fit into my pre-pregnancy clothes."

—Keri Hessel, Beautiful Babies student

"At the end of October 2012, I found myself lethargic, uninterested in most things, and frustrated with my weight. Most of all, I was disappointed that my husband and I had not conceived, even though we had been trying for over six months. Tracking my ovulation didn't seem to help.

When I ran across Kristen's website, Food Renegade, a week later, I immediately signed up for her free e-mail course on Beautiful Babies. Who doesn't want a beautiful baby?

I made little changes at first, then bigger ones as I found reliable sources for real, traditional food. My energy went up, my digestive issues stopped, and it felt like my brain worked again for the first time in years.

Best of all, a few days after Christmas, the home pregnancy test I took showed positive. I am eight weeks into my pregnancy with no nausea, enough energy to keep up with my three kids and two dogs, almost no mood swings, and the joy of anticipating a healthy pregnancy for myself and my baby."

—Robin Fuentes, Beautiful Babies student

With Heartfelt Thanks

"If you want to go fast, go alone. If you want to go far, go together."
~**African Proverb**

I do not stand alone, but on the shoulders of giants. So many have pioneered the way before me, and I am deeply grateful for the paths they forged, the research they amassed, and the voices they contributed to my journey.

In particular, I want to extend thanks to the Weston A. Price Foundation and its president Sally Fallon Morell, who introduced me to the concept of traditional foods and ancestral eating. The foundation has been pivotal in preserving and continuing the work of Dr. Weston A. Price, and I am thankful for their diligence growing a movement that is far bigger than any one of us.

I am grateful, too, for author, speaker, and farmer Joel Salatin, who not only wrote a moving foreword for this book, but has also inspired so many to embrace a model of pasture-based, sustainable agriculture that can literally save the world. Thanks go to journalist and author Michael Pollan as well, as his book, *The Omnivore's Dilemma,* not only introduced me to Joel's adventures at Polyface Farm, but inspired me to turn my passion for food and nutrition into a viable income for my family at www.foodrenegade.com.

I also need to extend special thanks to Dr. Cate Shanahan, whose book *Deep Nutrition: Why Your Genes Need Traditional Food* gave me a vocabulary for expressing how nutrition can have such a dramatic and powerful impact on our children's health and that of future generations.

I am grateful for all those who ushered this book along in ways both large and small—my husband, my friends, my mother, my students, my blogging peers in Village Green Network, my editors at Victory Belt Publishing, and so many more.

And finally, I am thankful for you, my readers. You not only keep my family fed, sheltered, and clothed, you keep me on my toes with your pointed questions and insightful comments!

This book is dedicated to GG Dada, my grandmother who reposed in the Lord this past year. She was an amazing wife, mother, and grandmother who showered us with her love by filling our bellies with hearty food and our hearts with happy memories. May her memory be eternal!

Foreword
by Joel Salatin

One of my favorite children's stories is *The Little Red Hen*, whose refrain "I'll do it myself" is a heartwarming lesson in self-reliance. In our modern high-tech culture accustomed to dependence on experts, segregated specialists, and celebrated victimhood, we should probably all revisit that famous children's story.

Rather than embracing self-reliance and personal responsibility, American culture worships fear and helplessness. For example, too many young people aspiring to farm spend their time filling out government grant proposals and hoping a bureaucrat will help them. Rather than step out in entrepreneurial risk fueled by passion and perseverance, they wait for an anointing from a charitable entity. I always tell them, "Just do it. Why wait?"

If three decades ago I had waited for someone else's nod of approval, financial or emotional, Polyface Farm would not exist today, and four generations of Salatins would not be living happily on our family farm. I didn't know much then. But I knew enough to start: movement creates movement. Seldom does the whole journey show itself; normally we can see only the first step. After taking that one, the next one becomes apparent. The question is not "What do you plan to do?" but "What are you doing now?"

One of the most common questions people ask me after a presentation is, "What can I do?" A corollary is, "What will it take to move our culture from apathy to action?" The growing awareness that modern American culture is birthing a disconcerting future begs for answers.

How do we curb autism? How do we pay for medical care in a civilization that leads the world, both now and historically, in leading chronic ailments? Cancer, heart disease, obesity, type 2 diabetes: In a century, we've exchanged a 98 percent mortality rate from infectious disease for a 98 percent mortality rate from chronic disease—the so-called Western problems.

Wouldn't you think that a culture clever enough to develop indoor plumbing, sewage piping, stainless steel, domestic electrification, and the motor car would be able to keep itself at least as free from chronic disease as the most undeveloped country in Africa? Really? I know someone will say that we have to die of something, that once infectious diseases were conquered, thanks primarily to sanitation and clean water, chronic disease would get us. The leading cause of death among women through the nineteenth century was infection caused by burns—hoop skirts and hearth cooking were a deadly duo.

Morbidity data does not support the notion that diabetes and heart disease eventually get the old-timers in more primitive societies. In other cultures, the people who do not succumb to infectious disease live longer than Americans, and they do it without chronic Western diseases. Why? The reason is that modern developed Western cultures are conducting the largest experiment in human history. We're the first civilization to ever routinely eat unpronounceable food. Food that you can't make in your kitchen. Animals raised as drug addicts, confined without fresh air and sunshine in giant fecal factories. Food that won't rot. Ever see a squirt of Velveeta cheese grow mold? If it won't rot, it won't digest.

We're the first civilization to grow food on land fertilized with acidulated, petroleum-enhanced chemicals. For the first time, we've broken through the genetic boundaries imposed by compatible sexual plumbing and created strange, promiscuous life forms called genetically modified organisms. As a society, we've abandoned our kitchens for the soccer fields. We're far more passionate about, and interested in, the latest Hollywood celebrity-bellybutton piercing than about what will become flesh of our flesh and bone of our bone at the dinner table.

Taken in aggregate, this massive experiment on the fuel for our internal community of three trillion bacteria is the riskiest game ever played in human history. In the face of this, what's a mother to do? Do we look at our little ones, wringing our hands on the way to ballet practice, to the Dilbert cubicle, feeling helpless and disempowered? What can I do?

We need Wonder Woman. I don't mean the one on TV. I mean Grandma! I mean that self-reliant gal whose meals cured us, whose smells captivated us, whose nurturing comforted us. We've practically lost a generation during our collective love affair with McDonald's, Stouffer's frozen dinners, Top Ramen, and Cheerios. We need to rediscover the secret to Grandma's good humor, wholesome soups, and soul-satisfying meals.

Enter *Beautiful Babies*. In this fast-paced, well-footnoted little tome, Kristen Michaelis gives us answers to the question: "What can I do?" With three children of her own and a huge fan base for her blog (Food Renegade), Kristen dares to take on the dietary dysfunction of our day. Armed with heritage wisdom, the latest science, and a healthy dose of faith in the way

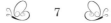

ecology and nature work, she gives the hands that rock the cradle a can-do recipe for success.

Want to virtually stop doctor visits? Want families with vibrant countenances like the ones adorning packages of Little Debbie's poison? Those kids didn't grow up on Little Debbie's. No, indeed. They grew up on butter, lard, pastured meats and poultry, copious amounts of eggs, and fresh vegetables. They didn't grow up on Pop-Tarts or muffins or Coke or Mountain Dew. Their parents didn't grab dinner in a bucket or bag from a drive-thru window.

This is a mom book. It's written by a mom for moms. One heart to another. It's a take charge thing. It's not about waiting for the American Heart Association to come around. It's not about waiting for the government to adjust healthy American dietary guidelines. It has nothing to do with recommendations from the American Medical Association, or what your insurance company will cover. Have you ever seen a mother hen fight for her chicks? She'll fight to the death to keep the hawk away. She'll fight a snake, a dog. Ever watch a cow defend her calf against a coyote? She'll die of exhaustion before letting a predator attack her calf. Kristen exhibits that spirit. Goodness, too many moms today have lost their protective instinct. They've formed alliances with the Coyote Association. Tragically, they don't think they're strong enough to fight the coyotes.

I find Kristen's feisty spirit and mischievous humor both empowering and liberating. I don't know how many men will read this book, but if you're a man and your precious partner is anxious about what to do, give this book to her right now. As a dad of two, husband of one, and grandfather of three, I covet these historically proven and normal principles for every family on earth. I wish this book had been around when my wife, Teresa, and I were starting our family. I can tell you one thing—I wouldn't have wanted to be the one to cross this mother. A lioness, indeed.

Fortunately, we were blessed with beautiful babies. We never bought baby food. Teresa breast-fed all our children—we never owned a bottle or bought an ounce of formula. We grew our own food or bought unprocessed local food. We always said that if we could grow toilet paper and facial tissue, we could pretty much pull the plug on society. Our kids played outside, never had a TV or video games, did chores, and have still never had a dental cavity.

I remember a couple of ear infections. Garlic drops worked fine. Home school. Family meals. Eating dirt outside. Building dams in the creek. Raising animals and growing a garden. Who needed the doctor? Some would say we were just lucky. But Teresa and I came from farming genetics. Both of us grew up drinking raw milk and churning butter. Our families had an unbroken chain of pickles, canning, and backyard gardening. Our children grew up in the same house I grew up in. Talk about tribalism. Hear my primal scream? Don't chop that vine—I'm swinging on it. Ha!

While I'm extremely grateful for healthy, happy kids and grandkids, I'm more grateful for a family of moms that took their role seriously, trusted in historical normalcy, and asked their grandmothers, rather than doctors, for advice. We definitely had some birthing complications, but we didn't have all of Kristen's guidelines to follow. I wish we had. We thought we were doing really well to not eat TV dinners and Velveeta cheese.

The nutritional body of knowledge has grown considerably in the last 30 years, thanks in large part to the Weston A. Price Foundation.

The whole idea here is not to promise success, but to create a climate in which success has a better chance to germinate. Every seed won't sprout. But if you give it fertile soil, clean water, good temperature, it has a much better chance than if you leave it on a dry tabletop. The goal is a habitat that incubates health.

Here's my question: If you—Mom—don't start doing something now, who will? Which malady or sickness will finally make you pay attention? Surely the principles our family has espoused, and those illuminated in the pages of *Beautiful Babies*, are not a guarantee for perfection or sickness-free living. But they do reduce the risk. They're the way to bet. They're the horses that have been winning races throughout human history.

And thanks to Kristen's selfless, passionate, protective maternal spirit, these principles can build an immunological fortress around our precious kiddos. It doesn't mean an interloper will never scale the walls. But we can at least make his entrance difficult. We owe it to our children. We owe it to our peace of mind. Now prepare to be empowered.

part one

Nutrition for Fertility, Pregnancy, Breastfeeding, & Baby's First Foods

Are you struggling to get pregnant? Did you know infertility is a mostly modern problem? Successful traditional cultures rarely, if ever, experienced infertility. In the first part of this book, you will learn about the nutrient-rich diets that fertile populations around the world ate when preparing their bodies to conceive and give birth.

Do you want a beautiful birth? Nutrition matters! Study after study has proven it. Proper nutrition can reduce your chances of getting a C-section and help you bring your baby to full term with the least amount of personal discomfort.

Do you want your child to never have an ear infection? Never need glasses or contacts? Never need braces? Did you know that the way you eat when you're pregnant can either give your child a wide face with high cheekbones—or a narrow face without enough room for all his teeth or tonsils? Did you know that what you eat while pregnant can actually make a long-term difference in your child's health?

Do you want to know how to avoid morning sickness? Or cravings for junk foods? Or varicose veins? Or stretch marks? Or swelling? In this book, you'll learn how to prevent or minimize the effects of these and other pregnancy pitfalls with the right nutrition.

Chapter 1
Paradigm Shifts

I don't like being yelled at. A part of me cringes when I'm called offensive names, or when my judgment as a mom is questioned. I don't have a competitive bone in my body. And when conflict comes knocking, I shrivel up and withdraw to an inward place of relative passivity.

Unless I'm angry.

Then I'm like a tigress—all claws and teeth.

Thankfully, this aggressive side of me only rears its head in private around my *safe* people (you know, people who will always love me, like my husband). In public, I attempt to be more constructive, particularly in the realm of public discourse. So imagine my surprise when a simple Facebook comment engenders a slew of caustic commentary. All directed at me.

Apparently, I'm controversial.

Am I writing about politics and religion? Am I calling people egregious names?

Nah. I'm writing about what's for dinner. I'm sharing that my nine-month-old daughter eats spoonfuls of butter, barely cooked egg yolks, and whitefish roe.

The butter is from grass-fed cows. The egg yolks are from pastured hens. The whitefish roe is wild-caught.

To my way of thinking, this makes her meal particularly nutrient-dense. In other words, it makes it *healthy!* Yet to many other parents, her meal is evil regardless of how well it's sourced. *Egg yolks? Butter?* Do I *want* to give her a heart attack? Make her obese *for life?*

On the contrary, I want my little one to grow up to be robust, have vibrant health, never need glasses or braces, and never struggle with her weight.

I'm a thinking mom, and I've made an educated choice. Somehow I've connected the dots and decided that following conventional nutritional wisdom doesn't actually make us healthier: it makes us sicker.

Despite this being a controversial thing to say, I say it anyway. In public. I declare it in blog posts. I write about it on Facebook. I teach it in online classes. What can I say? I'm passionate.

I want to help people. I'm not a doctor or nutritionist. In fact, I have absolutely zero official certifications or fancy initials behind my name. I'm just a mom who likes to research. And write. And teach. I'm what my friends affectionately call a "nutrition geek."

I didn't always care so much about nutrition. My conversion happened when I became a mother. A friend showed me the documentary film *The Future of Food*. My first son was just a few months old at the time, sleeping in his bed.

"You won't regret this," my friend said, popping the DVD into the player. "You may not be able to look at food the same way, but you won't regret seeing it."

She was right. The documentary opened my eyes to the story behind where my food comes from. I, like most Americans, thought the story of my food began at my grocery store. Oh, I *knew* rationally that it came from farms and was passed through distributors and manufacturers and turned into the products on the shelves (which I then bought and ate). But I'd never given any thought to the state of agriculture in my country. I'd never thought about the real life of the farmers or how government subsidies could actually have effects that trickled down into my food choices.

The biggest story inside *The Future of Food* is that of the advent of genetically engineered crops. The most striking part for me, however, wasn't about genetically modified foods. What haunts me are two of the last scenes of the film.

A farm worker wearing what looks like a space suit walks along rows of strawberries, spraying them with some kind of pesticide. Clearly, the man must wear the suit to protect him from exposure to the harmful chemicals and toxins. Ominous music plays, and the scene cuts to a young child eating a ripe strawberry, red juice dribbling down his chin. My heart skips a beat.

Did that child really just ingest those noxious toxins? The same toxins that had required a man to *wear a space suit* in order to handle them?

Strawberries are one of the most pesticide-laden crops on the planet. Because of their thin skins, pitted texture, and fine cilia-like hairs, it's practically impossible to wash any pesticides, herbicides, or synthetic fertilizers off the fruit. Every year, the Environmental Working Group collects data on which crops contain the highest amount of pesticide residues, and strawberries consistently rank in the top three.

How could I feed this to my own child? How could I knowingly involve him in a vast experiment on human health by feeding him newfangled, chemically-coated foods that had only recently been introduced to our collective diets?

For the first time ever, I wanted to buy organic food. I wanted organic not because it's more environmentally friendly, or because I suddenly devel-

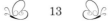

oped a social conscience. I wanted it because *until a hundred years ago, all food was organic.*

Think about that for a moment. We've been on this planet for about 200,000 years. Until about seventy years ago, all we ever had to eat was organic food. Now, in a few short generations, we've gone from having organic, whole food as the norm to chemically laden, genetically modified edible food-like substances as the norm. What would have been abnormal for almost all of human history is suddenly *normal*? Suddenly *healthier* than what has sustained us for millennia?

Being the geek that I am, I didn't want to be swayed by dramatic documentary imagery or romantic notions about human history. I wanted solid answers. I wanted knowledge that made intuitive sense. I wanted to learn from the wisdom of those who'd gone before me.

So, I stepped out of my normal food routines and into the shoes of what some might call a "food fanatic." I did my research. And I learned a *lot*. One thing I discovered is that everyone has their own idea of what "healthy" food is. Vegans, vegetarians, low-carbers, Dr. Oz. You. Me. And little of it is grounded in truth.

Consider where we get our ideas from. Many of us unconsciously absorb the not-so-subtle messages of food marketers, who go to great lengths to tell us how healthy their product is. They brandish their claims on their packaging, and in the ads they bombard us with on TV, the internet, and in magazines. These fill our minds with contradictory bits of data that leave us confused. To make matters worse, the so-called experts who are supposed to get it right—scientists who are working in the public interest and whose livelihoods don't depend on sales of particular brands of food—seem to change their minds frequently.

Remember when saturated fats were the devil incarnate? Every news article and television show gave the same advice: Avoid red meat! Chicken is king! Cholesterol is bad! Avoid eggs! My mother still has several behemoth tomes put out by the American Heart Association on a hundred and one ways to cook "heart healthy" chicken. But despite following all this advice as a nation, we still grew more obese and sickly.

In my own short life, I've seen fat *and* carbohydrates take significant hits. I've also seen little consensus in modern research. I've seen papers that argue against red meat on the grounds it increases heart attack risk while others argue *for* red meat on the grounds that it reduces heart attack risk because it's high in linoleic acid. I've seen studies that show that eating butter reduces the risk of coronary heart disease, while contradictory studies show that people who eat more butter risk dying prematurely from strokes.

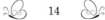

How can this be? How can we ever trust these so-called experts when they can't even agree with each other? And when they vacillate so much?

Here's what you need to realize. Our food "science" is relatively young.

As food journalist Michael Pollan says in his book *Food Rules*, current nutrition science is "sort of like where surgery was in 1690."[1] Think about that for a minute.

Nutrition science can help us understand why good food is good for us, but it cannot be the final arbiter of what is and is not healthy. The reason: simply because it's so *new*.

Not only is it new, but it's operating from the *wrong* premise. One of its biggest flaws is its tendency to reduce foods to their constituent parts—to single nutrients—and focus on the nutrients alone without considering their relationship to one another in pure, whole foods. That's shortsighted. A carrot is more than beta-carotene, a tomato more than lycopene.

As Nina Planck points out in *Real Food for Mother and Baby*:

> "[One] reason to eat whole foods is that many nutrients work together. Sperm health improves dramatically when vitamins A and E are eaten together, probably because E prevents oxidation of A. You need vitamin C to absorb iron, and saturated fats extend the use of omega-3 fats. There are countless relationships like this in nutrition. *There is no need to remember them. Just eat whole foods in their natural state and in classic combinations, such as leaves with olive oil, or fish with butter, and you'll get everything you need.*"[2]

The idea that individual nutrients matter most has led to an even bigger mistake, says Pollan: the idea that "with a judicious application of food science, fake foods can be made even more nutritious than the real thing."[3] Margarine is now considered "smarter" and "healthier" than butter. Milk made from genetically modified soybeans is touted as a healthier alternative to whole milk from cows. And where, exactly, has that thinking gotten us? Are we healthier? Or are we sicker and more obese?

The acceptance of the idea that food chemistry could improve upon nature marks a shift in our culture's dominant food paradigm. It didn't happen all at once, and there were those who fought hard against it. One such individual was Dr. William Khron, who published *Graded Lessons in Physiology & Hygiene* in 1901. (The book was used in Texas schools). I recently came across his book and thumbed through it for weeks, marveling at just how much common-sense knowledge we've lost when it comes to food and health. Dr. Khron's wisdom is striking, considering that he was probably

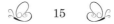

trained at the end of the nineteenth century, at a time when there were no real ways to monitor internal bodily functions.

In the book, Krohn is ardent in his defense of *real food*—a view shared by the culture at large. He wrote the textbook just at the time when margarine was undercutting butter and beginning to rapidly increase its market share, and only three years before vegetable shortening would do the same to lard.

This passage from the book says it all:

> "Many of our foods are sometimes spoiled by persons who manu-facture or sell them, putting into them cheaper substances that are dangerous to health. Such persons seem to care little for the purity of foods, but are chiefly interested in making the most money possible out of them. So common has this adulteration become that in most of the states the law-making power has passed pure-food bills to prevent the sale of such adulterated articles. These laws are most worthy and should be strictly enforced, for what is money-making by a few indi-viduals compared with the health of the people of an entire city or state, which may be greatly endangered by the use of these impure or adulterated foods?"[4]

In 1938, the widespread use of these phony foods caused the United States Congress to pass the Food, Drug, and Cosmetic Act, which required that the word "imitation" appear on *any food* that was an imitation. This law was in effect until 1973 when the food industry finally succeeded in getting the law tossed out.

Perhaps you're old enough to remember buying American cheese back when it was called "imitation cheese" instead of a "cheese food product." Maybe you remember seeing margarine labeled as "imitation butter" or jelly labeled as "imitation jam."

Not anymore.

Sadly, the foods Khron warned us against in the early twentieth century are accepted as commonplace today. They've been joined by an entire array of fake foods that line our grocery store shelves. To quote farmer and author Joel Salatin, most food products sold these days are "irradiated, amalgamated, prostituted, reconstituted, adulterated, modified, and artificially flavored, extruded, barcoded, unpronounceable things."[5]

Is that really what you want to feed your family? Do you really believe that's what's best for babies developing in the womb?

I want to return to an age when the dominant culture understood food as it did a mere hundred years ago. That's why I feed my daughter butter from grass-fed cows, egg yolks from pastured hens, and roe from wild-caught fish—as wise mothers have done in earlier times when we lived closer to nature and had a closer connection to our food. I believe that following the dietary wisdom of traditional cultures—which have kept people truly healthy and yes, beautiful for ages—makes more sense than slavishly following the dictates of modern nutritional science, which clearly has not kept people healthy.

Think about how long people have lived on this planet before the advent of industrialized farming and food production. Every native culture has had to grapple with the challenge of drawing sustenance from its environment. As a result, every native community has a highly developed food culture—with "rules" on what food to eat when, how to prepare and eat it, what to eat along with it, and what foods to avoid altogether.

These "rules" aren't arbitrary. They have arisen from the collective wisdom of the people. They reflect what people in that culture have observed about which foods and preparation techniques bring health and which cause illness, poisoning, or death. These traditional diets have kept people truly healthy for centuries, and because they have, they *ought* to be studied. Fortunately, they have been—and that wisdom is being passed forward by proponents of what has come to be called the "traditional foods" or "ancestral nutrition" movement.

My own study of these cultures has caused me to change everything I thought I knew about healthy eating. I've had my own paradigm shift. Now, I like to eat red meat. I think butter is good for me. I drink my milk raw. I avoid prepackaged foods like the plague. I don't believe the health claims on food labels. I like my food to be fresh, wholesome, and traditional.

In short, I choose *real food*. What is real food? At heart, it's the kind of food we ate before the industrialization of our food supply. This is food your great-grandmother would have recognized as food. This is the food that's been eaten for hundreds of generations on this planet. So simple, really! Most important of all, it's the wholesome, nutritious food that will not only give your baby the best start in life, but—as I explain later in the book—will help make sure that your baby is healthy enough to one day bear beautiful children of her own! Truly, the food choices you make while pregnant will influence not just the health of your own child, but of your grandchild and your great-grandchild, too. So choose wisely!

Chapter 2
Why Nutrition Matters

When people new to my little online kingdom stumble across one of my unconventional blog posts written in favor of a real food like butter, they often leave a sarcastic comment or two chiding me for my junk-food-loving ways. Dripping with derision, their words show me just how little they understood my point.

I'll never advocate that people eat junk food, particularly if that person is pregnant, nursing, or trying to conceive. That's because nutrition really does matter, possibly more than you might think. With every pregnancy, mothers-to-be are given this standard advice: Take prenatal vitamins. Avoid caffeine. Try not to eat too much junk. Avoid raw cheeses and cold lunchmeats. Don't drink alcohol.

Everyone knows nutrition matters.

But these bits of advice all tell us how to *avoid devastating deformities and abnormalities*. The prenatal vitamins are so that your baby doesn't get rickets or spina bifida. Avoiding alcohol keeps your baby's appearance and development normal by preventing fetal alcohol syndrome. Avoiding soft raw cheeses and cold lunchmeats protects you from contracting listeria and the host of potentially deadly problems that can accompany that disease in a pregnant mother.

Is it such a stretch to imagine that nutrition can do *more than just prevent these tragedies*? If really poor nutrition can cause the facial abnormalities associated with fetal alcohol syndrome, is it such a stretch to imagine that really excellent nutrition can cause perfectly proportioned faces?

Have you ever stopped to think about what a perfectly proportioned face could mean for your baby?

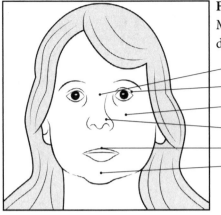

Fetal Alcohol Syndrome Face
Mother drank excessive alcohol during pregnancy.

low nasal bridge
small eye openings
flat cheeks

short nose & small sinus cavity
thin upper lip
recessed jaw

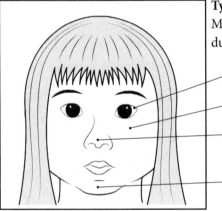

Typical Eskimo Face
Mother ate traditional fertility diet during pregnancy.

large, evenly spaced eye openings

wide, high cheekbones

well-proportioned nose & spacious sinus cavity

properly aligned jaw

Facial Structure	Implications
High cheekbones, wide dental arches	Plenty of room for all teeth. Everything grows in straight with no crowding. No need for braces!
Spacious sinus cavity	Plenty of room for drainage down the Eustachian tube. No ear infections, sinus infections, and fewer colds with less congestion!
Well-spaced eyes	Eyes grow to proper shape because they have plenty of room. This means no near- or far-sightedness. (No need for glasses!)

This is just the tip of the iceberg. Nutrition has far-reaching implications for fertility, your pregnancy and birth experience, and your child's long-term health.

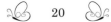

The Importance of Nutrition for Fertility

In 2007, a team of researchers at Harvard University found that women who consumed skim milk and low-fat dairy had 85% higher infertility rates than women who consumed whole-fat dairy.[1]

Despite this, how many women do you know who persist in eating a low-fat diet even when they're trying to get pregnant? How many women fail to realize the link between the amount of fat they eat and their hormone balance?

Hormones are made from cholesterol, and without adequate amounts of that in the diet (usually from fatty foods), our bodies can't make all the hormones they need. In short, without cholesterol, we'll suffer from hormone imbalance. Is it just me, or does that sound like the sort of thing that could keep you from getting pregnant? A low-fat diet is also associated with radically fluctuating blood sugar levels, which can also lead to a pregnancy-preventing hormone imbalance.

When I decided to let the diets of successful, traditional cultures guide me, I needed to find researchers who actually examined the anthropological evidence about what these cultures ate (for surely, it wasn't low-fat dairy). Only then could I understand what foods were prized, how they were prepared, and what foods were noticeably absent. Anything short of that would simply be my own romantic notions of history.

These days, it's hard to find cultures adhering strictly to their traditional diets. Virtually every culture the world over has been inundated with at least a few industrialized food products. The grandmothers in these cultures may claim to be making old-fashioned, traditional foods, but they're using modern ingredients that weren't even around a hundred years ago.

Perhaps they've replaced duck fat with canola oil, or are using refrigerated tofu instead of fermented tofu. Maybe they're no longer fermenting the grain for their flat breads like they used to, opting instead to mimic the sour taste with vinegar. Maybe they're buying their broths in cans or using MSG-laden bouillon instead of making a homemade broth from bones.

The exceptions to this rule are a few select, highly primitive, hunter-gatherer groups. Unfortunately, only a handful of researchers are studying them.

Even then, these cultures may not be called "successful." When I use that word, I'm describing a state of robust health, fertility, and aging with stamina. I don't want to know what malnourished, diseased people are eating. They're not models to follow.

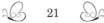

Rather, they are examples of diets that fail. I've already got plenty of examples of those. I just have to look around at my own culture with its epidemic rates of cancer, diabetes, heart disease, and obesity.

No, I want to look at what successful, traditional cultures had in common. What dietary choices tied them together?

For that, we can look at the work of Weston A. Price. A successful dentist and researcher, Dr. Price started the research institute of the National Dental Association. You may recognize this organization by its contemporary name—the American Dental Association.

Back in the 1920s, Dr. Price noticed an alarming pattern. More and more children were coming to his practice with dental deformities—cavities, overbites, narrow palates without enough room for the teeth to grow in straight.

He wondered why this was. Could it be genetic?

A quick look at their parents' and grandparents' perfect teeth and facial structure suggested not.

Perhaps it was related to diet? What did these kids eat that their own parents had not eaten?

A survey of their diets gleaned a list of likely suspects: refined white sugar, refined wheat flour, vegetable-based cooking oils, hot-water-bath and pressure-canned foods. These were all new on the American dietary scene.

Dr. Price hypothesized that these industrially produced foods were somehow lacking in the vitamins, minerals, and other nutrients our bodies need to create healthy teeth and bones.

To test his hypothesis, he needed to find cultures that were unaffected by dental decay or deformities. He would then test the foods they ate and compare the vitamin and mineral content to the modern American diet of his day.

Over the course of the next decade, Dr. Price traveled the globe and tested the diets of fourteen different successful, traditional cultures. His anthropological work was published in 1939 in *Nutrition and Physical Degeneration*.

He studied a wide variety of ethnic groups, including the Lotschental in Switzerland, the Inuit in Alaska, Polynesians on Pacific islands, Pygmies in Africa, Aborigines in Australia, and many others.

While their diets varied widely, they had many things in common. For example, all lacked industrialized food products like white flour, sugar, and vegetable cooking oils. All relied heavily on homemade bone broths. All relied heavily on some sort of fermentation process to help safely preserve food and ate a substantial amount of foods (particularly animal foods) in their raw or fermented states. Grains, if eaten, were soured with native bacteria or yeast, leavened through a natural fermentation process (like sourdough), or sprouted to make them more digestible.

But perhaps most telling of all is that when people within these societies strayed from their traditional diets and introduced even nominal amounts of industrially produced foods, they immediately showed signs of Western degenerative diseases.

It was when I was looking at the more than 15,000 photographs Dr. Price used to document his research that the tale he told really began hitting home. I saw photo after photo of healthy native people with wide, high cheekbones and perfect teeth. Each one of them ate a traditional diet free of industrialized foods. According to Dr. Price, they had perfect vision and were in prime health despite varying ages. Yet their beauty was all the more telling when contrasted against the narrow faces, pinched noses, and poor teeth of people from those same villages or tribes who had started eating white flour, sugar, and other industrialized foods.

Truly, a picture is worth a thousand words. Riveted by page after page of pictures, I became even firmer in my conviction that the path to health isn't along the road paved by government bureaucrats spouting the latest in nutritional dogma.

Rather, it can be found in the time-tested ways of growing, preparing, and eating food.

And how did these exceptionally healthy traditional cultures prepare their couples for childbearing?

In his study of healthy traditional people, Dr. Price observed that couples ate specialized preconception diets for anywhere from six months to a year before getting pregnant.

These diets were rich in a few key nutrients that radically increased fertility. They provided an optimal balance of nutrition for sustaining the health of mother, father, and infant.

Modern science has revealed that it takes nearly a hundred days for a woman's egg to mature before it is ovulated and seventy-two days for a man's sperm to form. This suggests that at the very least, a three-month period of optimal nutrition for a couple will produce the healthiest-possible egg and sperm.

So, why did couples in these traditional societies stretch out their fertility diets for six months to a year? It's been theorized that in a window of six to twelve months, the first half to three-quarters of that time was to help the body detox and heal, while the last three months promoted maximum fertility.

Oh, how the mighty have fallen. Does *anybody* these days follow a fertility diet for six months to a year before attempting to conceive?

Is it any wonder that one in seven couples is infertile (meaning they cannot conceive after a year or more of trying)?

Perhaps it's wrong of me to leap to conclusions about declining fertility rates in relation to our nutrient-starved diets. Yet I'm not alone.

Many studies have been done linking malnutrition with infertility. It is widely known, for example, that there is an association between malnourishment and amenorrhea (the abnormal lack of menstruation).

Numerous studies on cows, ewes, and other animals also show a definitive link between maternal nutrition and fertility.

When you think about it, it's really just common sense. Of course nutrition affects fertility. How could it not?

Perhaps the more controversial concept is that a modern American eating three meals a day could be malnourished. Yet, if Dr. Price's research showed us anything, it is that we are!

According to Dr. Price, traditional cultures placed a large emphasis on getting unique or special nutrient-rich foods for couples attempting to conceive. These foods fell into their own category and were considered sacred for their ability to promote life. For example, tribes who lived in the Andes mountain range would send men down to the sea to collect fish eggs they would bring back to their women. Hearty Gallic fishermen living on Scotland's coast would feed women of childbearing age a dish made of fish heads stuffed with oats and chopped fish liver. Hunter-gatherers in Canada, the Everglades, the Amazon, Australia, and Africa would save the liver, glands, blood, marrow, and adrenal glands of land animals for their wives.

When Dr. Price took samples of these preconception diets back to his lab for testing, he discovered they were particularly rich in the fat-soluble vitamins A, D, and K2. They were also high in folate, B6, and B12.

In many cases, people in traditional cultures consumed ten to twenty times more of these vitamins than the Americans of Price's day! Compared to these native fertility diets, our contemporary diet of industrially produced food is malnourished indeed.

Modern nutritional science has helped us unravel why traditional cultures may have placed such an emphasis on particular foods. It turns out that vitamin A is like the symphony conductor for pregnancy—without it an entire cascade of processes necessary for successful conception, pregnancy, and birth would go wrong. It is a nutrient the body needs to store in addition to being fed it regularly. You need vitamin A to make estrogen and the other pregnancy hormones that guide fetal development.

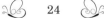

Recent studies on the connection between vitamin D levels and pregnancy found that women who had high blood serum levels of vitamin D reduced their risk of premature birth by half.[2] These women also saw a 25% reduction in infections, such as the cold and flu. Gestational diabetes, high-blood pressure, and pre-eclampsia were reduced by 30%. And babies born with the highest blood serum levels of vitamin D had fewer colds, less eczema, and were less likely to be considered "small." It's also important to note that vitamin D, in conjunction with healthy gut flora, is responsible for producing all the feel-good, "happy" hormones that will keep a pregnant woman's spirits up.

While much remains unknown regarding the role of vitamin K2 in a baby's development, we do know it is critical for making the myelin sheath on neurons in the developing brain, and it also greatly influences facial development. So, you want those high cheekbones and wide dental palates for your child? Eat a diet rich in K2.

We've also learned that deficiencies in the B vitamins, particularly B6 and B12, can cause infertility. Sadly, these are easily depleted when women use birth control pills, and without solid supplementation, B vitamins may take a long time to build back up in large enough quantities to produce a healthy baby. B12 is also essential for the male to create viable sperm, and men with low B12 levels have lower sperm counts.

Given the infancy of nutrition science, I'd be willing to bet there's even more to this story than meets the eye. These are just the nutrients Dr. Price knew of and that he thought to test for. Yet clearly, they all play absolutely vital roles in fertility and fetal development.

The Importance of Fetal Nutrition for Your Child

As it turns out, the roles of these essential nutrients may be far more extensive than originally imagined.

Dr. David Barker is both a physician and a professor of Clinical Epidemiology at the University of South Hampton in the UK. In 1989, he led a team of researchers in a study demonstrating that infants who had low birth weight ran a greater risk of developing heart disease later in life. It was the first time that well-known researchers tried to connect the dots between how a child developed within its mothers' womb and how that same child experienced either health or disease later in life.

Since then, Dr. Barker has published more than three hundred papers in scholarly journals and five books expanding on what has since been called "the Fetal Origins Hypothesis" or "the Barker Theory." What he and other researchers discovered is that foods eaten in pregnancy can significantly increase the baby's risk of contracting chronic diseases later in life. We're talking heart disease, high blood pressure, strokes, type 2 diabetes, obesity, osteoporosis, and more.

On October 4, 2010, the Fetal Origins Hypothesis made the cover of *Time* magazine. Journalist Annie Murphy Paul began that article with these words:

> "What makes us the way we are? Why are some people predisposed to be anxious, overweight, or asthmatic? How is it that some of us are prone to heart attacks, diabetes, or high blood pressure?

Paul listed the usual responses to these questions before saying this about the gist of the Fetal Origins Hypothesis:

> "But there's another powerful source of influence you may not have considered: your life as a fetus. The kind and quantity of nutrition you received in the womb; the pollutants, drugs, and infections you were exposed to during gestation; your mother's health, stress level, and state of mind while she was pregnant with you—all these factors shaped you as a baby and a child and continue to affect you to this day."[3]

Not long after that *Time* article came out, I was seated in a waiting room with a pregnant friend, watching as she read it. Maybe I imagined the weight of guilt settling over her, the shoulders drooping, and her shocked expression. Was she considering her own diet? Her own stressful life and how she was ruining her baby's future with each chocolate chip cookie she ate?

Maybe I imagined that. She was, after all, silent. Silent and reading.

But I didn't imagine the elderly gentleman next to us leaning toward her and commenting, "Shucks, ma'am. Don't you go worrying about that. Kids will turn out the way they turn out. You're puttin' too much responsibility on them shoulders of yours."

While he may have meant for his words to be kind, to ease a burden, they also rang hollow. The mother-to-be read the rest of the article. She became convinced—a believer.

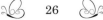

She learned, for example, about a pair of studies conducted at Harvard Medical School that found that the more weight a woman gained while pregnant, the higher the risk that her child would be overweight by age three and carry that extra weight into adolescence.

Of course, we could dismiss those findings as merely correlative. Perhaps the children shared the poor eating habits of the mother? Or possibly a genetic predisposition to obesity?

That type of critical thinking led Dr. John Kral, a professor of surgery and medicine at SUNY Downstate Medical Center in New York, to conduct a study comparing children born to obese mothers with their siblings born after the mothers had successfully undergone fat-reduction surgery. The younger siblings had similar genes to their older brothers and sisters, practiced similar eating habits, were raised in the same homes with similar stresses and identical socioeconomic backgrounds. The only real difference between the groups was that the younger children developed within non-obese mothers.

Those younger children? They were 52% less likely to be obese than siblings born to the same mother when she was still overweight.

How is this possible? Wouldn't genetics have more to do with it than this? Or the kind of diet the children ate?

In the last decade or so, more and more scientists have begun answering these questions using the theory of epigenetic modification through nutrition. (Try saying that three times fast!) *Epigenetics* is a fancy way of saying that nutrition or other environmental factors can influence the *behavior* of genes without actually altering DNA.

They talk about this in terms of genetic *expression*—whether or not a gene is turned "on" or "off" and expressed within the body. Many wrongly assume that genetics are written in stone, that once you're born and your genes are expressed there's no changing them.

Epigenetics disproves this. While the expression of some genes is unchanging once you're born, many others can change with dietary changes. What we eat as adults can change our current health and fitness levels, but we're limited. Once we're adults, for example, we can't change the shape of our face.

Genetics are most malleable when we're in the womb and in early childhood. That's yet one more reason why nutrition during pregnancy matters!

To silence, or turn off, undesirable genes, your body makes use of *methyl groups*. Your body gets the building blocks it needs to create these groups through methyl-donating nutrients like folic acid, B vitamins, choline, and SAM-e. Diets high in these methyl-donating nutrients can rapidly alter genetic expression, particularly when in utero and during early childhood development.

During these critical months, the *epigenome* (that genetic "on/off" tally sheet that influences which genes are active and expressed) is first being established. Dietary deficiencies in the methyl-donating nutrients can actually cause certain parts of the genome to be under-methylated for life.[4]

Translation? Those genes won't ever be easily turned on or off later in life. They'll tend to be stuck right where they're at, even if they're making you obese or creating heart disease.

The good news is that such change is not impossible, just harder. Studies have shown that adults who ate a methyl-deficient diet and experienced a decrease in DNA methylation could reverse this with the resumption of a methyl-rich diet.

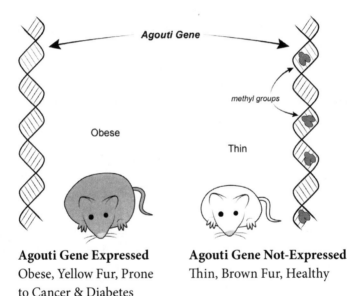

Agouti Gene Expressed
Obese, Yellow Fur, Prone
to Cancer & Diabetes

Agouti Gene Not-Expressed
Thin, Brown Fur, Healthy

In the figure above, you can see the results of a study shared in The University of Utah Genetic Science Learning Center's online guide to nutrition and epigenetics. Both mice are genetically the same, sharing a gene called "the agouti gene." When expressed, or "turned on," this gene causes the mice to be overweight and have yellow hair, and pregnant yellow-haired mice fed normal diets always give birth to yellow litters. Yet when they fed a methyl-rich diet to those mice during pregnancy, their litters were mostly healthy and brown—and remained so into adulthood! Do you see what happened? The agouti gene was

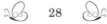

"turned off" in the pups, despite being "turned on" in the mothers—all because of better prenatal nutrition[5]

Both of these mice carry the Agouti Gene. Both had mothers who did not express the gene, and both had mothers who were fed BisephenolA (BPA) during pregnancy.

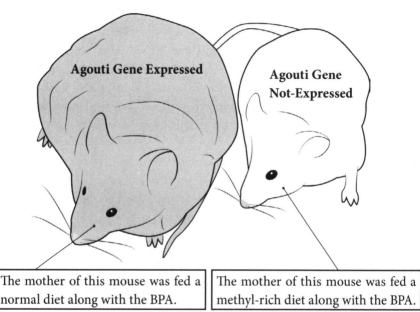

Agouti Gene Expressed

Agouti Gene Not-Expressed

| The mother of this mouse was fed a normal diet along with the BPA. | The mother of this mouse was fed a methyl-rich diet along with the BPA. |

Proper prenatal nutrition even protected the mice against the negative effective of Bisphenol A (BPA), a compound found to cause developmental abnormalities during early fetal development. Bisphenol A is used to make plastic.[6]

These mice suggest that what your mother ate when pregnant with you helped determine your genetic expression. Arguably, the tie can go back even further.

Did you know that the egg you grew from was created inside your maternal grandmother's womb when she was pregnant with your mother? It's such a wild thought!

But, it's true. Baby girls are born with all the eggs they will ever have. Unlike males, who can produce sperm throughout life, females don't create new eggs. Rather, the eggs they received in their mothers' wombs mature and are spent in a repeating cycle of fertility until a woman no longer has viable eggs. She may still have hundreds or thousands remaining, but they are no longer sensitive to follicle stimulating hormone, which is what causes the egg cells to mature into a viable egg. Menopause occurs naturally when a woman runs out of viable eggs.

So, not only is your epigenetic makeup determined by what your mother ate when pregnant with you, but also by what *her* mother ate when pregnant with *her*!

Dr. Cate Shanahan, author of *Deep Nutrition: Why Your Genes Need Traditional Food*, likes to call this "genetic momentum." We all inherit a particular genetic momentum from the generations gone before us. Did your parents eat a nutrient-dense diet? Their parents? If yes, then you've got a lot of genetic momentum going for you! You could probably be a lot more lenient with your diet and experience no ill effects until much later in life, if at all.

But what if your parents had poorer nutrition, and their parents, and so forth? What if you were born with a genetic momentum that was more like genetic inertia?

Dr. Shanahan has seen this often in her practice—a place where she has the opportunity to interact with families that span four generations at once. She has seen the eighty-five-year-old great-grandmothers who were born on family farms and retain perfect vision and teeth despite their age. And she has seen their great-grandchildren who have narrow jaws, frequent infections, and already need corrective eyewear despite their youth.

It led her to observe, "Today so many of us are sick ourselves that we've grown to accept disease as one of life's inevitables—even for our children. Today's kids aren't healthy. But rather than make such a sweeping and terrifying declaration, we avert our eyes from the growing mound of evidence, fill the next set of prescriptions, and expand our definition of normal childhood health to encompass all manner of medical intervention." To what does she attribute the degenerative changes? Poor diet—for at least three generations—coupled with "overconsumption of sugar and new, artificial fats found in vegetable oils." The end result, she says, may well be couples who are incapable of conceiving children at all.[7]

Such a scary prognosis! Say it ain't so.

Unfortunately, the evidence to back up Dr. Shanahan's personal observations is all around us. The Mayo Clinic reports that 15% of all American couples are infertile.[8] While no major studies have been done in the U.S. to verify whether infertility rates for couples here are rising, such studies have been done in other developed countries. For example, in Canada, the infertility rates in couples with a female partner between the age of 18 and 29 went up to 13.7% in 2009 compared to just 5% in 1984.[9] This is bad news for young couples, who are typically among the most fertile population age group.

Yet it's not just about rising infertility rates. Our children are sick, and will be sicker within their lifetimes than we ever were. In 2003, a study published in the *Journal of the American Medical Association* found that the lifetime risk of contracting diabetes for boys born in the year 2000 was 32.8%. For girls, the risk was even higher at 38.5%![10]

Can you imagine? Two out of every five girls born that year will contract diabetes!

And, according to the National Cancer Institute, the news is worse in regard to cancer. 41% of all children born in 2012 will be diagnosed with cancer within their lifetimes.[11]

This level of poor health ought to terrify us.

But instead of being scared into action, we grow fatter, sicker, and lament the "healthcare crisis" and "obesity epidemic." Yes, it is a crisis. It is an epidemic. But those word choices shuffle the blame off of *us* and make it sound like something being imposed from somewhere beyond, something completely outside the realm of our control. This type of language prompted Michael Pollan to tell Oprah, "When you hear the phrase 'healthcare crisis' or 'healthcare cost crisis,' that is a euphemism for the catastrophe that is the American diet."[12]

So what is the bottom line here? *There are a growing number of people with dwindling genetic momentum.* Each generation in their family has gotten progressively sicker, experiencing illness at a younger and younger age.

Clearly, nutrition matters.

You may have come into this life with a lot of genetic hurdles, but that doesn't mean you should give up! It took decades, and possibly lifetimes, to give you the genetic momentum you currently have. Should you be surprised that it might take years, even decades, of eating nutrient-dense foods to reverse that momentum before you see radical changes?

The authentically good news here is that your nutrition now is an investment in future generations—your children, your children's children.

So what does that nutrient-dense diet look like? Particularly when you're living in the modern, industrialized world?

Chapter 3

Just Say No

If we learned anything from the work of Dr. Price, it's that the single most important thing you can do for your health and wellness is to opt out of the industrialized food system altogether.

Unless you live on a farm, that's almost impossible to do. Many of us come close. We may shop at farmers' markets, buy directly from ranchers, and even attempt to cook most of our own food. But let's be reasonable; we all draw the line somewhere short of our ideal because we're living in the modern world.

We constantly encounter situations in which we must choose. How do I handle the snacks my child is provided at daycare? Do I insist on preparing my own snacks for my little ones? What if their caregiver is choosing healthier, but not ideal options?

My boys go to a community Bible study program each week. The teachers there adore the kids, and they don't want to feed the children sugary snacks. But their definition of sugary and my definition of sugary often conflict. Do I object to the organic graham crackers, apples, and orange juice? Or do I shrug my shoulders and try not to create conflict where none is really necessary? After all, it's not like my kids have any food intolerances or digestive issues that require a certain diet. Rather, I just prefer certain more nutrient-dense-foods over their less-nutritious alternatives.

What do we do when we're invited to dinner at a friend's house? Again, we have no real food intolerances. So, should I abstain from eating their macaroni and cheese, mashed potatoes, and steak just because it all came out of the industrialized food system? That steak isn't from a grass-fed cow. That cheese isn't from a local, pasture-based dairy. Do I lecture my friends (politely)?

What should I do when we're at church or a party? When we're traveling long distances and on the road? When we're in a hurry and too tired to have planned ahead? When we're visiting family on holidays?

For myself, I try to follow the 80/20 rule. If 80% of the food I feed my family is as nutrient-dense as I can afford, then I don't sweat the remaining 20% of the food we eat when at friends' homes or at social functions.

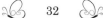

No matter where you currently draw your line, you need to pay careful attention to this chapter. Much of the information may seem old hat, but I've found that I can't skip it and assume that everyone has already mastered it all. Even when people know the dangers inherent in industrial foods, many have blind spots. And even if you've got no blind spots, you could probably use the extra motivation to move past some of your old stumbling blocks.

There's an inside joke among us card-carrying challengers of politically correct nutrition. We call the typical diet of the typical person eating modern industrialized foods (including junk food, fast food, and even the usual grocery store fare) "S.A.D." That stands for the Standard American Diet, and it is a sad diet indeed.

If you consider that we humans have been nourishing ourselves and our families for thousands of generations, the past hundred years of industrial food production are a tiny, barely significant blip in the continuum of history. Seen in this light, virtually every industrialized food is experimental. We have no idea what the long-term effects of these so-called foods will be on our bodies or how they'll affect future generations. Given our own observations, the growing weight of scientific research, and the anthropological evidence of researchers like Dr. Weston A. Price, we can make a pretty good guess, though. These foods are dangerous—for our health, for the environment, for animals.

In this chapter, I'm attempting the impossible. I'm trying to capture the highlights of just about everything that's wrong with industrialized food production. There are so many avenues to explore, and I'm not even going to walk down them all.

While this may seem like old news to many of you, it's been my experience that you can't just leave a discussion like this out of a conversation on eating for fertility, pregnancy, breastfeeding, or a baby's first foods.

Why's that?

Because it's not enough to just start eating foods that promote fertility and health. Many industrial foods actually repress fertility (like soy and MSG). Even many so-called health foods (like flax) counter fertility and pregnancy hormones. Plus, when people say they've eliminated processed foods from their diet, I've found that means different things to different people. For some, it means they gave up diet sodas in favor of real-sugar-sweetened ones. For others, it means absolutely nothing (and I mean *nothing*) goes into their bodies that they did not themselves cook from scratch. For yet others, it means they stopped eating fast food and buying potato chips, but still eat boxed whole-grain cereals in the morning with 2% milk.

Hopefully, my ramblings will provide some clarity. Even if you feel like you've covered this ground before, you never know what you might learn!

First Things First

When beginning any major lifestyle change, you have to learn to give yourself grace. Making real, lasting changes in our life for the better is hard work! So how can we go about it without becoming overwhelmed and discouraged?

This question was the basis of *What About Bob?*, a hilarious comedy released in the '90's that starred Bill Murray. In it, a successful psychiatrist writes a famous book called *Baby Steps*. Bill Murray plays Bob, an overly dependent psychiatric patient who tries to implement these baby steps to create lasting social and psychological improvements in his life.

Although the idea of taking baby steps is the butt of many jokes in the film, the concept, in truth, is not without merit. *Any* changes you can make, no matter how small, *do* make a difference.

In Japan, it's called *kaizen*. It's a strategy for making change based on tiny, continuous improvements. And they *do* mean tiny. Want to build a habit of exercise? A *kaizen* practitioner would recommend you start by marching in place for one minute a day. The point is to make changes in small but effective increments. You start with where you're at, and you look to see what you can change. You make it your goal to change that one thing.

Then, you give yourself grace. Lots of grace. Grace to break *every other rule*. You work on your one thing—and only that—until it's habitual.

Every diet adjustment, even the simplest, takes time. It may be two, three, or even four months before you're comfortable in your new eating habit—before it "fits" like an old pair of boots. But it *will* happen. And once it does, you can evaluate where you're at and make another small change.

With time, you'll have made dramatic and sweeping changes to your diet—changes you would have scoffed at as impossible merely a year ago.

So consider this my advice: remember *kaizen*. Make one change at a time and *master* that change. *Own it.* Then move on to the next. You won't regret it.

Saying No to MSG and Other Additives

In 1908, the Japanese isolated monosodium glutamate (MSG) to enhance food flavors, particularly meat-like flavors. Did you know we actually have glutamate receptors on our tongues? It's the protein in food that the human body recognizes as meat. The invention of MSG meant that just about any protein could be hydrolyzed to create free glutamic acid—meaning that there was now a way to create intense, meat-like flavors without any meat present.

To get those flavors before the invention of MSG, people the world over used bone broths. Now industry had created a way to shortcut the lengthy and nourishing process of creating stocks from the bones of beef, chicken, lamb, pork, and fish. They could make food that tasted "just as good" at a fraction of the cost.

But at what cost to our health?

Research on the dangers of MSG continues to mount, albeit slowly. Some contend that funding for such projects is inevitably sparse. After all, why would the food industry (which funds most of these sorts of research ventures) want to spend money proving the detrimental effects of one of its chief money makers?

There are a growing number of people who report immediate, adverse reactions to eating MSG. Perhaps you're one of those people. Or maybe you know someone who is sensitive. Complaints include burning sensations in the mouth, head, and neck; weakness of the arms or legs; headaches and upset stomach within minutes of consuming MSG.[1] Some people even describe getting heart palpitations and hives or other allergic skin reactions.[2]

"Wait!" you say. "I call foul. How do they know what these people experienced was actually because of eating MSG? How were these experiments controlled? Were they double-blind? That's the only real way to do epidemiological research like this."

It's true that when people self-report what they're eating or how they're feeling, their own bias tends to get in the way. They misremember exactly what they ate. They make associations between what they consumed and how they think they *ought* to feel. But double blind studies on the effects of MSG have been done. These are studies where neither the participants nor the people administering the study know who consumed MSG. Everything's randomized and controlled by researchers a step removed from the process. And guess what? Even these double-blind studies found that MSG exposure caused muscle tightness, fatigue, numbness or tingling, and flushing in sensitive people.[3]

But what if you're not one of those people? What if MSG causes no noticeable or immediate reaction in you? Should you still consider it a dangerous food additive?

Yes!

That's because the effects of MSG are cumulative. Just because you don't react to MSG now doesn't mean you won't later. According to Dr. Russell Blaylock, who wrote a book on the subject called *Excitotoxins: The Taste That Kills,* sensitivity to MSG builds up in our bodies until we reach what he calls our "threshold of sensitivity." That's because MSG overstimulates the nervous system—exciting the nerves and causing an inflammatory response. With time, these repetitive, inflammatory responses cause our nerves to produce more and more nerve cells that are sensitive to this kind of stimulation. The more overly sensitive nerve cells we have, the stronger our immediate response to MSG will be.[4]

That said, you still might be scratching your head about MSG. If the worst that can happen is a migraine headache or some hives, why worry about eating it now, when it causes no reaction in you?

Way back in 1957, a team of researchers decided to see if glutamate could help repair a diseased retina. Remember, glutamate is a common and necessary amino acid in our diet (also one of the most common neurotransmitters in the brain), so this presupposition isn't so far-fetched. The researchers fed rats MSG and were shocked by their results.

Rather than repairing the disease, the MSG destroyed the retinal cells that allow vision.

A decade later, the neuroscientist Dr. John Olney used their method of destroying retinal cells so that he could study visual pathways to the brain. He found that MSG not only destroyed retinal vision cells, but also parts of the brain. This brain damage was done as neurons became over excited, virtually exciting themselves to death. He called this "excitotoxicity," and that has led subsequent researchers to describe MSG as an "excitotoxin."

While the naturally occurring glutamates in food aren't dangerous, processed free glutamic acids like MSG are.

Not only do they cause brain damage and lead to nervous disorders, but they also cause radical hormone fluctuations. Mice injected with MSG rapidly become obese and inactive, and develop other hormonal issues.[5]

"Wait!" you say. "Those are mice and rats. We're people. We're bigger, biologically different. Surely it won't affect us the same way."

Unfortunately, that argument doesn't hold much weight. Humans are twenty times more sensitive to MSG than monkeys, and five times more sensitive to it than rats.[6] We have glutamate receptors on every major organ,

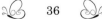

hardwired into our brain, and even on the tip of our tongue! That means that one fifth the level of MSG used to cause obvious brain damage to a rat will do the same to you.

And what about growing babies? It turns out that MSG is especially harmful to pregnant or nursing mothers because infants and young children are four times more sensitive to MSG than adults![7] According to Dr. Blaylock, "many studies have shown that glutamate plays a major role" in brain formation during fetal development. The developing child's brain is exquisitely sensitive to any oscillation in brain glutamate levels. Too high levels of MSG in the mother's diet during pregnancy may put child at greater risk for developing learning disabilities, behavioral and emotional problems, addictions, and endocrine disorders.[8]

I don't know about you, but this is enough for me to raise alarm bells. Not only is MSG not a traditional food, not only are many people immediately sensitive to it, but it can also interrupt the hormonal and biological development of my children!

Lest you think this is all fanciful, remember that a number of studies report that MSG's effects can occur cumulatively over time with subsequent exposure. For example, a study done with animals found that MSG exposure over a period of three to six months led to significant risk of damage to the retinas of the eyes.[9] Initially, there was no visible damage, but multiple exposures over a period of time led to the irreparable injury.

It's simply not worth the risk.

So if you want to avoid MSG, how can you do it? Turns out, it's harder than it looks.

If all you had to do was read food product labels and put anything that said "monosodium glutamate" back on the shelf, you could maybe avoid MSG without too much difficulty. Or, if you could trust a food manufacturer's claim that there is "No MSG Added" to their food, that would make things relatively simple, too.

But MSG hides in more than forty FDA-approved ingredients. Because the manufacturer didn't add an ingredient called "monosodium glutamate," they can "truthfully" claim "No MSG Added" on their label. Yet nothing is stopping them from adding ingredients that *contain* MSG. In that case, the manufacturer only has to list the name of the actual ingredient added, *not the ingredients within those ingredients.*

So, they can say a food includes "spices" or "flavorings" when that spice mix includes MSG. They can say the food includes "yeast extract" or "hydrolized soy protein" without telling you that the process of creating those ingredients also creates processed free glutamic acids (also known as MSG).

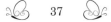

For more on where MSG may be hiding in your food labels, see Appendix A.

Of course, MSG is not the only dangerous additive in our food supply. There are other excitotoxins—like aspartame (found in NutraSweet and other artificial sweeteners) and L-cysteine (a common dough conditioner found in bread products).[10]

But beyond excitotoxins is an entire world of chemical or synthetic additives used to enhance the flavor, visual appeal, and shelf life of our foods. Are all these additives harmful or dangerous? Where the science is concerned, the jury is still out.

Some organizations, such as the Feingold Association (www.feingold. org), have compiled huge amounts of research on the potential risks and hazards of synthetic food coloring and other food additives. They've summarized a lot of this research on their website. They have found that the food dyes, Yellow # 5 and Yellow # 6, contain significantly more parts per billion (ppb) of benzidine, a known carcinogen, than the FDA allows. The allowable limit is one ppb; one small study of nearly 70 samples of Yellow # 6 showed that half contained as many as 10 ppd of benzidine, and one sample showed levels as high as 941 ppb.[11]

Even if you're not willing to believe these food additives are, in themselves, harmful, consider this.

The butter made from the milk of cows eating rapidly growing spring grass is *yellow,* taking on a bright *golden* hue at room temperature. Compare this with the white butter made from conventional milk. Eggs from hens eating green pasture and fresh bugs have *deep orange yolks.* Compare this with the pale yellow yolks of conventionally raised hens.

In nature, color equals nutrient density. We're hardwired to respond to color. That's why artificial colors play such a *huge* role in packaged, processed, industrial foods. I'm not just talking about neon-blue and purple breakfast cereals or the orange of Cheetos. Even seemingly benign foods are full of artificial colors to make them look appetizing. (Yes, I'm talking about the yellow-green of your pickles.) In a 2011 article in *The New York Times,* Kantha Shelke, a food chemist and spokeswoman for the Institute of Food Technologists, revealed that: "color often defines flavor in taste tests. When tasteless yellow coloring is added to vanilla pudding, consumers say it tastes like banana or lemon pudding. And when mango or lemon flavoring is added to white pudding, most consumers say that it tastes like vanilla pudding. Color creates a psychological expectation for a certain flavor that is often impossible to dislodge. Color can actually override the other parts of the eating experience."[12]

Isn't that amazing? We are so hardwired to respond to the color of our food that it *actually overrides the flavor of our food.* Our brains will literally reinterpret the true flavors present in light of the colors present!

Removing artificial colors will even make tasty, flavor-filled junk food tasteless. The same article also revealed that consumers given Cheetos Crunchy Cheese Flavored Snacks that did not have artificial orange color found the snack "bland." Without the color, "their brains did not register much Cheese flavor even though the Cheetos tasted just as they did with food coloring," said Brian Wansink, a professor at Cornell University and director of the University's Food and Brand Lab.[13]

So I have a question for you. If the color of food is that important to our experience of taste, then *why would we ever want to eat food that **needs** to be artificially colored in order to be palatable?* Wouldn't that inherently mean that the food was total junk?

My homemade, naturally fermented pickles are naturally *green.* Yet store-bought, industrially jarred, vinegar-brined pickles are naturally *gray.* Shouldn't that tell us something? On the one hand, we've got a colorful, nutrient-dense, raw, living food. On the other, we've got a dead, cooked, nutrient-empty, edible food-like substance that needs food dyes to be added so we can stomach its vinegary flavors. Which would you prefer?

For more on how to spot artificial food colorings and sweeteners in your food, read Appendix A.

Saying No to Corn Derivatives and Corn-Fed-Animal Foods

I once spent a summer in rural Mexico, teaching Spanish to the children of an indigenous tribe. During that summer, I felt like I only ever had three meals. Corn tortillas and beans. Corn tortillas, beans, and chicken. Corn tortillas, beans, and goat.

Every morning, before dawn slipped over the mountains, while the stars still shined brightly in the sky, the village women would line up at the mill. Turned by a donkey, the giant slab of stone rotated around, grinding corn. The women carried the day's corn to the mill in buckets, all shucked and removed from the cob, and soaking in a mixture of water and the mineral lime. The mill rooster would crow. The donkeys would bray. The goats could be heard bleating. The sounds carried through the mountain valley like a tidal wave of wakeful energy. The village came to life when the mill did,

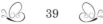

grinding their soaked corn into a sticky corn-flour paste that they flattened and cooked to make tortillas.

I never needed an alarm clock.

Corn is the backbone of that tribe's diet, supplemented with beans, goats, chickens, and a variety of vegetables like tomatoes, squash, and peppers.

I honestly don't want to knock corn. When traditionally prepared, the grain is rich in vitamins and can easily fill the belly, leaving you sated and healthy.

Yet corn has sadly become overabundant in our industrialized food world. We don't just grow it to feed ourselves; we grow it to feed our animals. And then we strip it apart in laboratories to create a cocktail of food additives like high-fructose corn syrup and maltodextrin.

If you find a corn-derived ingredient on your food label, chances are excellent that you're eating a food that's too industrialized and processed to be healthy.

To understand some of the risk in the overconsumption of corn, you first have to know a bit about essential fatty acids.

There are two families of essential fatty acids (EFAs): omega-3 fats (sometimes called "n-3") and omega-6 fats (sometimes called "n-6"). These fats are *polyunsaturated fatty acids* (PUFAs), and they serve some amazing purposes within our bodies. We use them to help regulate cellular inflammation, moods, behavior, signaling between cells, and many other cellular functions.

The most important thing science has learned about omega-3 and omega-6 fats is that their ratio to each other in our diet can cause a cascade of biological responses in us—everything from inflammation (which can lead to heart disease or diabetes) to mood swings.

In the traditional diets studied by Dr. Price, the ratio of omega-6 to omega-3 fats was roughly anywhere between 4:1 and 1:4:[14]

- Hunter-gatherers living mostly on land animals: 2:1 to 4:1
- Pacific islanders getting most of their fat from coconut and fish: 1:2
- Inuit and other Pacific Coast Americans: 1:4 or less
- Dairy-based cultures: 1:1 to 2:1
- Cultures eating fish and grains: 1:2 or less

This also roughly correlates with contemporary findings on the ideal ratio of omega-6 to omega-3 fats in the diet. In an article for the *American Journal of Clinical Nutrition*, scientists summarized worldwide research by

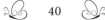

saying, "The World Health Organization/Food and Agriculture Organization suggests a ratio of 5:1 to 10:1, Sweden recommends a ratio of 5:1, Canada recommends 4:1to10:1, and Japan recently changed its recommendation from 4:1 to 2:1."[15]

The science everywhere agrees that when the ratio of omega-6 fats to omega-3 fats gets too high, the results are unhealthy:[16]

- Inflammation of the arteries increases. This, in turn, promotes arterial buildup of cholesterol. The excess cholesterol clogs the arteries, increasing blood pressure and the risk of heart attack or stroke.

- Moods become volatile, tending toward depression and anxiety.

- Behavior patterns change, leaning toward low-energy levels and insomnia.

- Basic cellular functions are interrupted.

In the standard modern diet of industrialized foods, the typical ratio of omega-6 to omega-3 fatty acids is 20:1! That's because industrialized food production has become *dependent on corn,* which has an omega-6 to omega-3 ratio of 46:1.

Maybe you don't think you eat that much corn, but you may be surprised where it's hiding. Not only is corn in obvious places like corn tortilla chips or popcorn, but it's also hidden in manufactured and processed foods in the form of various corn derivatives. It's also fed to most industrialized animals, including cows, chickens, pigs, goats, ducks, and various kinds of farmed fish or seafood.

As Michael Pollan notes in *The Omnivore's Dilemma,* corn is in more than a quarter of the forty-five thousand items in the typical grocery store. Its chemical derivatives include:

- Modified or unmodified food starch

- Glucose syrup

- Maltodextrin

- Crystalline fructose

- Ascorbic acid

- Lecithin

- Dextrose

- Lactic acid

- Lysine

- Maltose

- High-fructose corn syrup

- Caramel color

- Xanthan gum[17]

In these forms, corn is in your coffee creamer, canned fruit, bread, ketchup, soups, and cake mixes. It is in your mayonnaise, hot dogs, and salad dressings. It is even in non-food items like toothpaste, diapers, and trash bags.[18]

Why has industrialized food production been so inundated with corn? Because it's cheap.

Why is it cheap? Because back in the late 1970s, the U.S. government decided to start subsidizing corn production. The government pays farmers to grow corn. This encourages farmers to grow corn even when they couldn't otherwise make any money doing it, even when there's no demand for it. So, every year since then, the U.S. has had a surplus of corn.

With so much extra corn floating around, it makes corn artificially cheap. Rather than grazing cows on grass, it's cheaper for a farmer to feed them corn. Rather than using sugar, it's cheaper for a food manufacturer to use high-fructose corn syrup. You get the idea. Of course, the cheaper a food is to produce, the more profitable it becomes to the company making it.

This excess of corn has caused the vast majority of foods created by industrial food production and growing methods to be unnaturally high in omega-6 fatty acids. And, as you read earlier, excessive dietary intake of omega-6s is one of the primary causes of heart disease.

But beyond chronic diseases, recent studies suggest an imbalanced omega-6 to omega-3 ratio is likely responsible for lower sperm counts and male infertility.[19] Considering how easy it is to have an imbalanced essential fatty acid ratio if you're eating the Standard American Diet, it only makes sense that couples seeking to get pregnant should weed out exorbitant omega-6 fats from their diet.

Later in this chapter, we'll talk about how to avoid the excessive omega-6 fatty acids found in modern, refined vegetable oils and foods from industrially raised animals. To learn how to avoid corn derivatives in food products, be sure to read Appendix A.

Just Say No to GMOs

You've heard of GMO crops, haven't you? GMOs (genetically modified organisms) are crops that have been substantially altered using genetic engineering. They're unnaturally modified foods whose safety is dubious at best. Europe, Austria, France, Germany, Greece, Italy, Luxembourg, Norway, the UK, Portugal, and Spain all have bans on GM crops.

Unfortunately, they're extremely pervasive here in America. In 2011, 94% of the soybeans grown in the U.S. were genetically modified, as was a whopping 88% of the corn.[20] These crops were sold to farmers around the world by a handful of mammoth biotech corporations promising radical yield increases.

According to a 2009 report published by the Union of Concerned Scientists, those promises are empty. While it's true that we've seen crop-yield increases in the fifteen years since the use of GMOs became widespread, the report argues that other factors led to those increases. In fact, when they contrasted yields of genetically engineered soybeans to organic yields for soybeans, the organic crop outperformed the GM crop by 13%.[21]

But the fact that GMO crops fail to live up to expectations and to the biotech industry's promises is almost irrelevant compared with the environmental and health risks associated with these crops.

If you had to name the largest single threat to the environment you could think of, what would it be? Climate change? Deforestation? Overpopulation? Wars? Pollution? A global pandemic?

My answer is easy: The single greatest threat to our planet is the presence of genetically modified organisms (GMOs) in our food supply. Decimate our food supply, and the rest won't matter. But are GMOs really *that* dangerous? Yes!

And here's why: GMO crops cross-contaminate. That means non-GMO corn planted in a field next to genetically engineered (GE) corn will take on the GE characteristics in its next generation.

So if there's anything—*anything*—remotely unsafe or undesirable about a GMO crop, it can spread like wildfire through our food supply.

Take, for example, a frightening genetic mutation currently being investigated by biotech firms. It's ominously called the "terminator gene." The terminator gene is designed to render the seed and crop it produces sterile, giving such seeds the moniker "suicide seeds." The biotech firm Monsanto currently owns the patent on this gene, which has no agricultural or economic benefits for farmers or consumers. The only reason Monsanto has to use this gene is to protect their "intellectual property." If their genetically

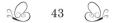

modified seeds can't reproduce, that <u>means the farmers who buy them have</u> <u>to repurchase seeds every year</u>, making Monsanto more money and giving them a monopoly on the market.

This may not sound so bad to you, but consider the law of unintended consequences. Remember that many GMO crops have already been shown to transfer their patented genes to wild relatives or similar, but non-GMO crops. Cross-pollination is a natural part of the world. So <u>imagine for a mo-ment what would happen if this suicide gene were to cross-contaminate other plants?</u>

A *Discover Magazine* article summarized it like this: "The scope of the problem is unimaginably vast: More than one billion people rely on saved seed in developing countries each year. Two-thirds of the population of sub-Saharan Africa subsist on small, low-production farms."[22] What would happen if those farmers suddenly found that the seeds they saved to feed their families were suddenly sterile?

Speaking of undesirable genes in GMO crops, have you heard of *pharm-ing*? It's the use of GMOs to manufacture pharmaceutical compounds.

Most scientists cheer the effort on, particularly the pharming of ani-mals. After all, you can get as much antithrombin (a protein found in human blood plasma and now manufactured into the milk of GMO goats) from a single GMO goat in a year as can be derived from ninety thousand blood donations.[23]

When you're talking about a single, well-protected herd of two hundred goats producing amounts of pharmaceutical proteins equivalent to those in eighteen *million* blood donations, the risks seem minimal.

After all, the goats are sheltered from the outside world. They're carefully bred under strict laboratory conditions. The chance of the mutated GMO goat milk making its way into our food supply is almost nil.

But what about other forms of pharming?

<u>Pharming plants poses an altogether different set of risks. Unlike ani-mals, where breeding can be closely monitored, plants tend to breed with the work of the wind, bees, or birds.</u> Cross-contamination between non-GMO and GMO plants is notoriously hard to prevent, despite the best precautions.

Since the wind alone can carry corn pollen for miles, it's not hard to imagine a pharmaceutical-laced GMO corn plant spreading its genes to a nearby cornfield growing corn meant for human consumption. We'd be eating dangerous, physician-prescribed pharmaceuticals in our cornflakes and not even know it.

Drugs currently being manufactured in crops include (but are not lim-ited to):

- vaccines for cholera, anthrax, plague, influenza, hepatitis C, lymphoma, and other deadly diseases
- interferon for liver diseases
- spermicidal antibodies
- insulin[24]

The thought of unintentionally ingesting any of these pharmaceuticals should give us all the willies.

But aren't GMO crops safe? Surely, they wouldn't be planted in open fields if there was any real risk of us getting sick, would they?

After all, if they weren't safe, they wouldn't be FDA-approved, right? After the massive recalls in recent years of peanut butter, spinach, cookie dough, and other foods, that question is almost laughable. But here's an answer for you: There has been almost no testing done on the safety of GMOs—none.

They were passed through the FDA by giant agribusiness lobbyists arguing that GMOs aren't substantially different from their non-GMO counterparts. In other words, it was just an argument. Just words. *There weren't actual clinical trials done on the safety of GMOs.*

And the few trials that *have been* done have shown alarming results—allergies, increased cancer risks, damaged food quality. Many GMOs are created using antibiotic-resistant genes, and the British Medical Association cited this as one reason GMOs should be banned worldwide: they pose a threat for the future efficacy of antibiotics.[25]

A 2009 document prepared by scientists in the EU summarized some of the scarier studies done on the safety of GMOs and found:

- Rats fed GM tomatoes developed stomach ulcerations[26]
- Liver, pancreas, and testes function was disturbed in mice fed GM soy[27] [28] [29]
- GM peas caused allergic reactions in mice[30]
- Rats fed GM rapeseed developed enlarged livers, often a sign of toxicity[31]
- GM potatoes fed to rats caused excessive growth of the lining of the gut similar to a pre-cancerous condition[32] [33]
- Rats fed insecticide-producing GM maize grew more slowly, suffered problems with liver and kidney function, and showed higher levels of certain fats in their blood[34]

- Rats fed GM insecticide-producing maize over three generations suffered damage to liver and kidneys and showed alterations in blood biochemistry[35]

- Old and young mice fed with GM insecticide-producing maize showed a marked disturbance in immune-system cell populations and in biochemical activity[36]

- Mice fed GM insecticide-producing maize over four generations showed a buildup of abnormal structural changes in various organs (liver, spleen, pancreas), major changes in the pattern of gene function in the gut, reflecting disturbances in the chemistry of this organ system (such as in cholesterol production, protein production, and breakdown), and, most significantly, reduced fertility[37]

- Mice fed GM soy over their entire lifetime (24 months) showed more acute signs of ageing in their liver[38]

- Rabbits fed GM soy showed enzyme function disturbances in kidney and heart[39]

But wait! It gets worse.

Here in the U.S., GMOs in your food aren't required to be labeled.

That means that even if you had an allergic reaction to a GMO, you'd have no way of knowing that the GMO crop caused it. In other words, the public health effects of GMOs are currently untraceable.

Why should you care? Because if you're an American and you consume corn and soy products that are not explicitly labeled "organic" or "GMO free," chances are you're eating these foods! Actually, it's an 80% chance, because according to current estimates, *80% of the food available in your grocery store contains GMOs!* [40] The most common genetically modified crops are corn, soybeans, cottonseed, canola (rape), sugar beets, and papaya. Considering how many processed foods contain soy, corn, canola, and sugar, coupled with the high saturation of GMOs throughout these crops, that's not surprising. But isn't it highly alarming?

Biotech corporations are vehemently opposed to the idea of labeling GMOs. Why?

Because they know if GMO products were forced to be labeled (as they were in Europe), consumers would stop buying them. Right now, these products are all pervasive and most people don't even know they're eating GMOs. If they saw the GMO ingredients in their tortillas, their cookies, their infant formula, they'd think twice about buying them.

As should you!

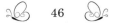

Saying No to Modern Vegetable Oils

Next to olive oil, the cooking oil marketed as the most "heart healthy" out there is canola oil. But what is it?

Canola oil is a newly created oil, invented in the 1970s as a low-erucic-acid version of the otherwise not-really-edible rapeseed oil. In 1998, through the marvels of genetic engineering, the now ubiquitous variety of rapeseed (which makes up roughly 87% of all rapeseed grown in the US and Canada) was created. So, it's safe to say that almost all nonorganic varieties of canola oil come from these genetically modified plants.

But what about organic canola oil? This comes from a naturally selected, low-erucic-acid rapeseed plant. But even though it doesn't originate in genetically modified plants, the oil itself is still unhealthy. That's partly because canola oil is between 28 and 35% polyunsaturated fats. In traditional food cultures, polyunsaturated fat intake made up less than 4% of the total calories eaten.[41] If it isn't good for traditional cultures, neither is it good for us.

And according to Mary Enig, Ph.D. (author of *Know Your Fats: The Complete Primer for Understanding the Nutrition of Fats, Oils, and Cholesterol*), "Although the Canadian government lists the trans fat content of canola at a minimal 0.2%, research at the University of Florida at Gainesville found trans fat levels as high as 4.6% in commercial liquid canola oil."[42] Trans fats indisputably increase risk for coronary heart disease, and a 2007 study found that for each 2% increase in the intake of energy from trans fats, women experienced a 73% greater risk of ovulatory infertility.[43]

How did those trans fats get in there? Because of how this oil has to be made. You see, prior to the Industrial Revolution, making seed-based cooking oils was *far too labor intensive* and, in many cases, downright impossible. All the ancient cooking oils (like coconut oil, palm oil, olive oil, and so forth) are easily pressed out of the plant without needing extremely high pressure or high temperature extraction.

After the Industrial Revolution, we had the technology necessary to create modern, seed-based cooking oils. So we did.

But the process of making and refining these oils translates into one thing: *rancid polyunsaturated fatty acids* (PUFAs). PUFAs don't hold up well under heat or pressure. The same is true for almost all modern, vegetable-seed-based cooking oils. Soybean oil is roughly 58% polyunsaturated fatty

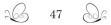 47

acids—nearly twice that of canola! Corn oil is 55%. Peanut oil is 32%. Sunflower, 40%. So, in the process of being extracted from the seed, these oils oxidize, and many of them plasticize (turn into trans fats). The end result is stinky and unappetizing, so the oil is further "cleaned" using bleach or alternative chemicals to deodorize it.

Gross!

And we call this heart-healthy?

And even if these high levels of PUFA weren't a concern, you would still need to be alarmed at the high ratios of omega-6 to omega-3 fats found in these modern, refined cooking oils. According to the National Nutrient Database released by the United States Department of Agriculture, corn oil has an omega-6 to omega-3 ratio of 54:1, and soybean oil of 54:7.[44] Even safflower oil—which is often touted as a "healthy oil" (like olive oil) because of its high percentage of monounsaturated fats—has an undesirable omega-6 to omega-3 ratio of 13:1.

Furthermore, safflower oil is like all industrially produced modern oils in that its edible form wasn't possible until the invention of modern extraction methods. Yes, a variety of safflower oil is indeed ancient, but the ancient methods of creating it made it suitable only for use in paints! It wasn't until 1925 that modern, industrial methods of extracting oil from seeds made it possible to extract *edible* oil from the safflower plant. I should say, "so-called edible."

The organic and natural food industries want to capitalize on your desire to eat quality fats. So they often sell organic versions of these seed-based oils and claim they are "expeller pressed." This mysterious-sounding term simply means that the oil wasn't extracted with a heated chemical solvent like hexane. Rather, the soybeans, corn, rapeseeds, and other seeds were heated, then put under extreme pressure to release the oil. While this process is free of chemicals, it is still going to create rancid PUFAs.

The bottom line is this: You need to avoid modern, refined vegetable oils.

Avoiding these oils may be harder than you think. Sure, you can choose to cook with other oils. But these yellow-seed-based oils are in just about every processed food available at your supermarket. You'll have to start reading ingredients labels if you truly want to avoid them. Furthermore, most restaurants and fast food chains cook with these oils. While you may not be able to completely avoid these oils when eating out, you can avoid exposing yourself to them by not ordering foods cooked in oils, particularly at the high temperatures that cause the delicate PUFAs to oxidize. Translation: Avoid foods fried in yellow-seed-based oils (items such as French fries, fried chicken, or tortilla chips).

Saying No to Industrial Meat

When I was a child, red meat was demonized. Everyone knew eating well meant eating chicken—lots of chicken. "Heart healthy" cookbooks cropped up everywhere, each one full of the same advice.

Of course, these days, science has shown us that the original lipid hypothesis—the idea that eating saturated fat and cholesterol leads to heart disease—is simply false. (More on that in Chapter 7!)

We now know, for example, that our bodies use cholesterol to heal and repair damage to our cell walls. Simply because cholesterol is present at the site of the injury doesn't mean it's responsible for the harm done. It's like saying our white blood cells cause infection, when in fact they are our body's defense mechanism to fight infection and keep it at bay. Because most cell-wall damage happens in the form of inflammation (which can lead to atherosclerosis, the hardening of the arteries), you can think of cholesterol as a team of firemen. They're on the scene to *put out the fire*, and are not themselves responsible for the fire.

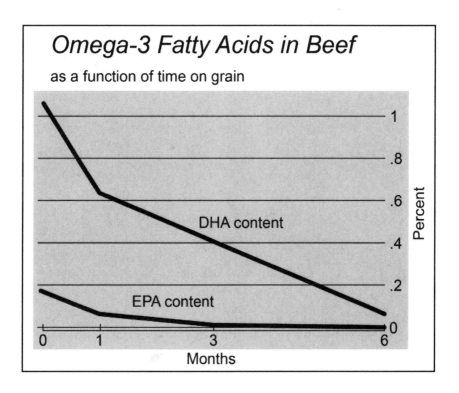

Omega-3 Fatty Acids in Beef

as a function of time on grain

So if we don't need to fear the saturated fat in meat, what do we need to fear? How can we tell which meat is unhealthy and which meat is actually good for us?

According to the research of Dr. Bill Lands, a nutritional biochemist and an authority on essential fatty acids, we want to keep our polyunsaturated fat intake below 4% of total calories, and we want an omega-6 to omega-3 ratio no greater than 4:1.[45]

That right there eliminates almost all industrially raised meats. You won't be surprised to learn that a cow fed a diet of corn has an omega-6 to omega-3 ratio of roughly 21:1! Similar statistics are found for pigs, chickens, and even farm-raised fish.

Notice in the graph above that just six months of feeding grain (think: corn, soy, and silage) to a cow is enough to dramatically reduce the omega-3 content of the beef to almost zero. So the standard practice of raising cattle on pasture and transferring them to a Concentrated Animal Feeding Operation (CAFO) for the last six months of their life to "fatten them up" makes the meat quite unhealthy for us.

The same thing happens in just about any CAFO—even those raising seafood.

Besides the abnormal fat content of industrialized meat, there are a host of other problems that make it less than ideal.

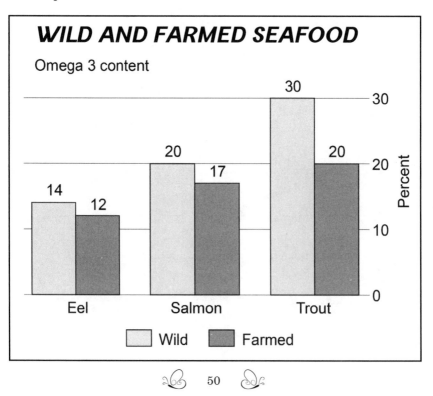

WILD AND FARMED SEAFOOD

Omega 3 content

Have you ever been to a Concentrated Animal Feeding Operation? Even know what it is?

It's a factory farm—an industrial facility—used for finishing livestock, including cows, pigs, chickens, and turkeys, prior to slaughter. Ninety percent of hogs and 97% of poultry live their entire lives on factory farms in the United States.[46] Ninety-six percent of all cattle finish their life in a CAFO.

The CAFO's primary goal? To make the most amount of meat in the shortest amount of time. It's about efficiency.

Don't go to a CAFO. Even if you're daring. Even if you're brave. You won't be able to stomach it.

The awful stench is the ammonia and hydrogen sulfide gases—toxic air pollutants directly responsible for the death of farm workers who enter poorly ventilated manure-containment systems. According to the Pew Commission on Industrial Farm and Animal Production, CAFO "facilities can be harmful to workers, neighbors, and even those living far from the facilities through air and water pollution, and via the spread of disease. Workers in and neighbors of [these] facilities experience high levels of respiratory problems, including asthma."[47]

No wonder. The waste from one cow is more than twenty times the waste of a human. Multiply that by 10,000 cows all confined to a small space, and you have the waste of a small city of 200,000 people on your hands.

But it's more than the smell, more than the pollution of our air, soil, and water. Factory farmed meat comes from some of the sickliest and most disease-infested animals on our planet, animals with compromised immune systems, animals so sensitive to illness that they're fed a steady diet of antibiotics. Humans who need to go near them must don space suits. (Technically, they're called bioprotective suits.)

I'm not making this up.

According to the Pew Health Group, "Up to 70% of U.S. antibiotics go to animals raised on industrial farms that aren't sick, to offset crowding and poor sanitation. This practice promotes the development of deadly strains of drug-resistant bacteria that can spread to humans. Penicillins, tetracyclines, macrolides, sulfonamides, and other antibiotics intended for humans are typically premixed in poultry and livestock feed or added to drinking water, often giving food animals constant low doses of antibiotics over much of their entire lives."[48] Is it any surprise that antibiotic-resistant bacteria cost the U.S. healthcare system an estimated $4 billion to $5 billion per year? [49]

On top of all this, the grain-based diet these animals eat is unnatural, and it produces unnatural meats. Cows, for example, are ruminants. That means they eat grass. Not grains. Grass. Their bodies were created to metabolize grass and turn it into meat. In a typical CAFO, cows are fed a diet of grains; chicken manure; dead animal parts; waste products from food, beverage, and candy factories; and silage. No grass is to be found. Anywhere. This industrial diet makes the cows sick because it aggravates and imbalances their digestive acids and enzymes, making their bodies acidic and disease-prone.[50] And their sickness passes to humans.

Consider the *E. coli* bacteria. Normally *E. coli* is a harmless part of our normal gut flora. Until relatively recently, *E. coli* infections in humans were rare. That's because almost all the strains of the bacteria that might have made us sick could not survive our stomach acids. However, an acid-resistant strain, E. coli 0157:H7, developed as an adaptation to the overly acidic stomach of the modern, grain-fed cow.[51] Now able to withstand the cow's more acidic stomach, the bacteria is also able to withstand our own stomach acids, making us ill.

Antibiotic-resistant bacteria. Unnaturally dangerous strains of otherwise common bugs. Sickly animals. Environmental devastation. Inhumane treatment of animals.

Hmmm … Industrial animal production is quickly amassing a long list of dire offenses. Is it any wonder I suggest you opt out of industrial meat production?

Saying No to Industrial Dairy

One of my friends, AnnMarie Michaels of www.cheeseslave.com, had the opportunity to tour a California dairy as part of a public relations tour meant to highlight the state's "happy cows." It was a family-owned industrial dairy. Cows lived in covered, open-air barns devoid of natural, vitamin-D-producing sunlight unless they were lined up to be milked or fed grains. They stood day in and day out on a concrete floor or mat covered in their own manure. They lay down in their own manure. They battled flies. Their average lifespan? Five years. The normal life of an unstressed dairy cow is closer to twenty.[52] And the stench! The smell was so strong it made my friend feel like throwing up.

In this scene, did you notice the rolling green hills of tall, swaying grass? The idyllic blue sky and sunshine? The quaint red milking barn? The happy cows standing in the pasture, slowly munching on their grassy food?

Neither did I.

The picture painted for us on food marketing labels is false.

Surely you know a handful of people who are dairy-intolerant. As with any food intolerance, the symptoms range from digestive problems to mood swings. And like gluten intolerance, dairy intolerance is rapidly on the rise. People aren't just on gluten-free diets. They're on casein-free diets (casein being the primary protein found in milk).

It doesn't surprise me. Modern, industrial milk is notoriously hard to digest. On so many levels, it hardly resembles traditional milk at all.

What's wrong with industrial milk?

Most industrial milk comes from more recent breeds of cattle producing milk abnormally high in A1 beta casein. A1 beta casein is a slightly different milk protein than the ancestral one common to more traditional breeds of cattle, sheep, goats, and even humans, known as A2 beta casein. Mountains of scientific research have been done on the subject of A1 beta casein, the way our bodies digest it, and the slew of mental and physical disorders it can cause.[53]

Most industrial milk comes from cows fed a disproportionate amount of grains. The most nourishing milk comes from cows being fed their natural diet of grass—the greener, the better. We'll discuss this more in the next chapter.

Most industrial milk is pasteurized. What is pasteurization? I'm glad you asked. It's a quick heat process designed to kill unpleasant bacteria and protect us against infectious diseases. But it does not guarantee cleanliness. Every single outbreak of salmonella from contaminated milk in recent decades has occurred in *pasteurized* milk—milk that's supposed to be "clean."

Besides not being the fail-proof protector we're told it is, pasteurization does a lot to rob milk of its value as a source of good nutrition. From Sally Fallon's *Nourishing Traditions*, we read this succinct summary of the pasteurization process:

"Heat alters milk's amino acids lysine and tyrosine, making the whole complex of proteins less available; it promotes rancidity of unsaturated fatty acids and destruction of vitamins. Vitamin C loss in pasteurization usually exceeds 50%; loss of other water-soluble vitamins can run as high as 80%; the Wulzen or anti-stiffness factor is totally destroyed as is vitamin B–12, needed for healthy blood and a properly functioning nervous system. Pasteurization reduces the availability of milk's mineral components, such as calcium, chloride, magnesium, phosphorus, potassium, sodium, and sulfur, as well as many trace minerals. There is some evidence that pasteurization alters lactose, making it more readily absorbable. This, and the fact that pasteurized milk puts an unnecessary strain on the pancreas to produce digestive enzymes, may explain why milk consumption in civilized societies has been linked with diabetes.

"Last but not least, pasteurization destroys all the enzymes in milk—in fact, the test for successful pasteurization is absence of enzymes. These enzymes help the body assimilate all bodybuilding factors, including calcium. That is why those who drink pasteurized milk may suffer from osteoporosis. Lipase in raw milk helps the body digest and utilize butterfat …

"Modern pasteurized milk, devoid of its enzyme content, puts an enormous strain on the body's digestive mechanism. In the elderly, and those with milk intolerance or inherited weaknesses of digestion, this milk passes through not fully digested and can build up around the tiny villi of the small intestine, preventing the absorption of vital nutrients and promoting the uptake of toxic substances. The result is allergies, chronic fatigue, and a host of degenerative diseases." [54]

Most industrial milk is homogenized. Homogenization is a process whereby all the fat molecules are mechanically forced to be the same size. (With homogenized milk, the cream doesn't separate to the top and is dispersed throughout.) Unlike pasteurization, no debate is underway on any purported health benefits of homogenization. But there are many sound reasons to *distrust* homogenization, such as the huge increase in surface area on the fat globules. The original fat-globule membrane is lost and a new one is formed that incorporates a much greater portion of casein and whey proteins, potentially leading to milk-related allergies. [55]

Most industrial milk is adulterated. After pasteurization, they add back in fat-soluble vitamins (like vitamin D) in a synthetic and arguably indigestible form. Without the usable and *real* vitamin D, the body can't make good use of the calcium in milk. If the milk has fat removed (as in skim, 1%, and 2% varieties), it's not only going to be missing all the fat-soluble vitamins the body needs to properly digest the calcium and other goodies in the milk, but it will also usually have nonfat dry milk or other milk solids added to create a more desirable consistency. These forms of dry milk are high in free glutamic acids (also known as "MSG") and oxidized cholesterol (a dangerous, inflammatory form of cholesterol that can cause heart disorders). [56]

Most industrial milk contains pus. Because modern dairy cows have been bred to produce up to four times as much milk as a traditional cow did a mere century ago, they are far more prone to mastitis: infected udders. If the mastitis gets out of control, the cow is temporarily removed from the herd and treated with antibiotics. When it finishes its course of treatment, the cow is allowed back into the herd. Some farmers cut corners, reinstating sickly cows before all the antibiotics have passed through the cow's system. The result? Antibiotics in your milk. Although that is initially a scary thought, it is actually quite rare in dairy cows.[57] I'm more concerned about the low-grade mastitis that goes untreated in industrially raised dairy cows. Farmers can get away with this because the FDA allows a whopping seven hundred fifty thousand somatic cells (more commonly known as "pus") per liter!

Much industrial milk contains synthetic growth hormones. Many dairy farmers give their cows rBGH or rBST, genetically engineered growth hormones designed to increase milk production. These hormones come out in the milk, you drink them, and then they play games with your own hormones, potentially leading to a number of problems, including infertility and cancer.[58]

Saying No to Industrial Eggs

Most of the eggs you can buy at your supermarket come from something called a "battery hen." Battery hens are laying hens that are born, raised, and spend the duration of their short lives in something called a "battery cage."

The earliest version of the battery cage was developed in the 1930s when agricultural enterprises wanted to emulate the newly discovered efficiency of factories by making farms factory-like. The cages were a runaway success, quickly overtaking the poultry industry. Battery cages are made of wire, allowing droppings and feathers to fall through the floor of the cage to a moving conveyor belt below. They also have a slanted floor designed to allow eggs to roll out of the cage and onto yet another conveyor belt that collects eggs.

As with all mechanical marvels, every need of the hen is taken care of. Food and water are delivered in set amounts at designated intervals to battery hens, using large conveyor systems. The feed often contains growth-promoting drugs like arsenic and antibiotics.[59] It may also be formulated with whatever vitamins and minerals are the latest health craze in an effort to boost that nutrient's content in the resulting eggs. Want more omega-3's? We'll deliver. Want some magical lutein? We've got it for ya! Vitamin B12, E, or B6? No problem.

We used to consider taking care of animals a form of "husbandry," a humane act of guardianship where we nurtured and protected animals from harm in exchange for the food they produced. Now, the process has been entirely mechanized, and any concern for the authentic health and safety of

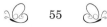

the hens has been stamped out. Baby roosters, of course, being useless to the operation, get routinely destroyed.

In perhaps the most deplorable feature of the battery cage, the ability of a chicken to express its natural inclinations—to behave like a chicken and enjoy its "chickenness"—has been thoroughly eradicated due to the radically small size of the cage and a life spent forever inside it. Most battery cages are barely larger than the hens they contain. Within weeks of hatching, hens are shuttled into the cramped cages. They then spend the next nine months unable to move or turn around—simply eating, pooping, laying eggs, and pecking at each other until they die.

The European Union banned battery cages in 2012, after a twelve-year phase-out that began when legislation was passed in 1999 against battery cages. They argued that the practice of raising hens in battery cages was inhumane. Particularly offensive were the routine removal of the hens' beaks, an activity necessitated by the stressed hens constantly attacking and pecking at each other. They also found the inevitable development of osteoporosis in battery hens equally reprehensible. Because movement and exercise in battery hens is so restricted, most hens cannot even walk (and can barely stand) on their fragile bones. Battery cages aren't just brutal, they're also unhealthy. Crowded conditions are a breeding ground for bacteria like salmonella, which can be transmitted through the eggs of the battery hens to the rest of us.

If you're at all conscientious about your food, you probably want to opt for something better than eggs laid by battery hens. But the other industrially raised options for eggs aren't much better.

These days, everyone's confused about what's actually humane and healthy when it comes to eggs. A case in point:

One day my friend dropped this little bomb in a conversation about how her husband and she navigate their food choices. "We've agreed to disagree about the kinds of eggs we buy. Whenever I go shopping, I buy the free-range kind. Whenever my husband goes, he buys the cheapest eggs he can find. I insist on buying the free-range eggs, because I know you say they're healthier."

"Ah, but really they're not," I say. "At least not when it comes to supermarket eggs."

Her smile quickly fades. "Oh."

You see, according to the law that governs labeling, "free-range" doesn't mean much of anything. What makes eggs healthy and nutrient-dense is hens having access to the outdoors, to sunlight, to bugs, and to grass. If a label says "free-range," it guarantees none of those things.

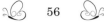

In fact, "free-range" can simply mean that hens have "access" to the outdoors. These hens are raised indoors from infancy and may not even choose to go outside. If and when they do, they may simply be walking out onto a concrete slab devoid of any nutrient-giving bugs, larvae, or grass.

A similar thing can be said for the "cage-free" label. All that means is that instead of being crammed into cages stacked on top of one another, hens are cage-free. They can still be confined indoors for their entire lives, never seeing a day of sunshine.

Even "organic" eggs only guarantee the chickens were fed organic feed and didn't receive antibiotics. They could still have limited or no access to the outdoors, and their diet is surely unnatural, being made up mostly of corn and soy.

Industrialized agriculture is no stranger to organic food. Sadly, organic standards in egg production do little to produce a nutrient-dense egg from an authentically happy hen. Industrial organic egg producers take advantage of the letter of the law to violate its spirit and cheat consumers out of hard-earned dollars by asking them to pay premium prices for eggs that are essentially the same as any other.

In 2010, the Cornucopia Institute released their definitive report on the subject. They call it: *Scrambled Eggs*.

One of my favorite zingers from the report:

> "Industrial-scale producers sometimes buy old conventional henhouses and convert them by taking out the cages. In order to meet the organic requirement for 'outdoor access,' they commonly build a small, insignificant concrete porch that is accessible through one or two small 'popholes.'
>
> "When they build new henhouses specifically for organic production, they do not move away from this model, but rather build very large barns housing many tens of thousands of chickens, with nothing more than a small concrete-covered porch as token outdoor access." [60]

And they call this "free-range"! Seriously, folks, you can't trust those supermarket labels. Here's another example of how Big-O Organic industrialized egg production violates the spirit of the "cage-free" label:

> "Aviary systems, allowing many more birds in individual buildings as compared to free-floor systems, are also popular with industrial-scale producers. Using this approach, houses can hold eighty-five thousand birds or more—examples are Herbruck's Poultry Ranch's

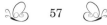

Green Meadows Farm in Michigan and Cal-Maine's new organic buildings in Kansas. According to one organic producer who specializes in pastured production, some types of aviary systems are, essentially, "glorified cages." Because cages are opened during the day, allowing the hens to roam freely on the floor, industrial-scale producers consider this a "cage-free" operation, and eligible for organic certification.

"In these aviaries, when the hens first move into the house, they are confined in multi-tiered cages. After some time, the doors to the cages are opened to allow the hens to access scratching areas on the floor of the house ... Those in cages on top levels have stairways to access the floor. Partitions divide the hens into flock sizes of 130 to 150 birds." [61]

"Well," you say, "perhaps that's *some* organic egg producers. But surely not the majority? Surely most farmers going for the organic label have a conscience?"

Nope. The report continues: "According to the United Egg Producers, a trade group for industrial-scale egg producers, and estimates by some producers, 80% of [organic] eggs come from the largest producers in the industry, with layer houses that mirror the conventional/industrial model of production and do not provide enough outdoor space for every hen to be outside at the same time."[62]

Put simply, everything about industrial egg production in this country—organic or not—is *ugly*. From the stench to the confinement, the crowded conditions to the mechanization. I think we ought to remember Wendell Berry's warning words, "If a thing is ugly, I think we need to ask questions about it. How did it get that way? What else is wrong?"

Just Say No to Refined Sweeteners

Everybody knows it. Sweets are bad for you. Yet even the healthiest among us keep coming back to them, making them a regular part of our daily eating habits. Why is that?

We're hardwired to like sweets. That's because in nature, sweet foods often come with a lot of other stuff that's good for us: dietary fiber, vitamins, and minerals.

Yet we live in a world full of unnaturally sweetened foods. Rather than telling us what food is ripe and full of the most nutrients, our sweet tooths are actually undermining our collective health. In 2008, researchers at Penn

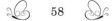

State determined that sugar is not only addictive, but that we need progressively more and more of it to satisfy our sugar cravings.[63] In other words, as you eat sweets, your tolerance for sweet foods increases. Eventually, you'll be adding twice as much sugar to your sweetened tea just to get it to "taste the same."

Refined sweeteners, usually in the form of table sugar or corn syrup, saturate the industrial food supply. Added sweetener is in just about every processed food, even things we don't think of as "sweet" like ketchup, beef jerky, mustard, mayonnaise, yogurt, bread, and salad dressings.

Your great-great-grandmother probably ate about five pounds of sugar a year. If you eat like the typical American, you're likely to eat that much in just two weeks![64]

While dehydrated sugarcane juice has been around for hundreds of years, the stuff we call sugar has not been. Not only is it often made from genetically modified sugar beets, but it is also a highly refined product of the Industrial Revolution.

In light of this, many people try to avoid eating refined sweeteners by switching to either artificial or natural alternatives. Since artificial sweeteners are completely new to the human diet and often untested for safety regarding long-term consumption, I cannot recommend them.

There was a time when people knew that eating sweets made them gain weight. In the last thirty years, we've switched our cultural emphasis away from the evils of sweets and onto the evils of fats. Only the growing popularity of the low-carb movement is shining any light on what used to be a commonly held truth: Eating refined sweets makes you fat. It's how our bodies are programmed to respond.

When you eat something sweet, your blood sugar level (the amount of glucose in your bloodstream) rises. Your pancreas then secretes insulin, a hormone that tells your liver to start taking up the glucose out of the blood and convert it to glycogen for storage in the liver. This, in turn, makes your liver stop transferring fat out of your adipose tissues (fat cells) and burning it for energy. Instead, your liver starts using its own stored glycogen reserves to fuel your cellular metabolism.

Did you catch that?

When you eat sugar, your body stops burning fat as a fuel source. If you eat a diet unnaturally high in refined sugars, you are training your body to expect a continuous influx of glucose. That means your body will rarely, if ever, have a blood sugar level low enough to require it to burn fat for energy.

What happens when you eat too much sugar? If your liver has already stored all the glucose it can in the form of glycogen, then your body converts the excess glucose into fat for storage in your fat cells.

Thus, a diet high in sugar trains your metabolism to stop burning fat for energy and to store excess energy as extra fat in your fat cells.

Not only that, the science regarding refined sugar is quite damning. Dr. Nancy Appleton compiled a long and glaring list of scientific studies done on the effects of eating refined sugar. Here are some of the more startling ones:

- Sugar can suppress your immune system and impair your defenses against infectious disease.[65]
- Sugar can cause a rapid rise of adrenaline. It can also give rise to hyper-activity, anxiety, difficulty concentrating, and crankiness in children.[66]
- Sugar can produce a significant rise in total cholesterol, triglycerides and bad cholesterol and a decrease in good cholesterol.[67 68 69 70]
- Sugar feeds cancer cells and has been connected with the development of cancer of the breast, ovaries, prostate, rectum, pancreas, biliary tract, lung, gallbladder and stomach.[71 72 73 74 75 76 77]
- Sugar can cause hormonal imbalances such as: increasing estrogen in men, exacerbating PMS and PCOS (poly-cystic ovarian syndrome), contributing to infertility, and decreasing growth hormone.[78 79 80 81 82]

Clearly, the excess refined sweetener in our diet has far-reaching ramifications. If you're hoping to increase your fertility and have a healthy pregnancy, just say no to refined sweeteners.

Just Say No to Synthetic Pesticides, Herbicides, and Fertilizers

The single most important factor in producing healthy vegetables and fruits is growing them in healthy, fertile soil. The farmer and prolific author Joel Salatin has said, "a culture can never be healthier than its soil."[83]

In *The Soil and Health*, Sir Albert Howard writes, "The soil is, as a matter of fact, full of living organisms. It is essential to conceive of it as something pulsating with life, not as a dead or inert mass. There could be no greater misconception than to regard the earth as dead: a handful of soil is teeming with life."[84]

Fertile soil is soil that is "teeming with life"—life that is born, dies, and breaks down in a never-ending cycle, creating soil that is rich in nutrients made readily available to the plants growing in that soil.

Unfortunately, modern agricultural practices have neglected the life and quality of the soil. Rather than creating rich soil teeming with life, industrialized agriculture has created dead soil inundated with synthetic fertilizers and pesticides. Not only is the food grown using these synthetic chemicals less nutrient-dense, it may also be dangerous for you.

But, before I get ahead of myself, I think it's important to first unpack the history of what synthetic fertilizers are and how they came into widespread use. You see, synthetic fertilizers rely heavily on three primary nutrients: nitrogen (N), phosphorus (P), and potassium (K).

These are the basic building blocks of plant life. Without them, a plant simply won't proliferate. But, in the same way that nutrition scientists want to think that we can understand human nutrition by looking at isolated nutrients rather than whole foods, plant scientists want to think that these three isolated nutrients are sufficient for plant life. Maybe I'm oversimplifying things, but the way that these scientists have heralded the N-P-K synthetic fertilizer as a powerhouse that will increase crop yield would be criminal if they seriously believed that soil needed to be nourished rather than plundered. Obviously, a plant's ecosystem is far more diverse and complex than a simple combination of N, P, & K.

In the *Fatal Harvest Reader*, farmer Jason McKenney describes how this kind of thinking is leading to the death of industrial soil:

"We now know that massive use of synthetic fertilizers to create artificial fertility has had a cascade of adverse effects on natural soil fertility and the entire soil system. Fertilizer application begins the destruction of soil biodiversity by diminishing the role of nitrogen-fixing bacteria and amplifying the role of everything that feeds on nitrogen. These feeders then speed up the decomposition of organic matter and humus. As organic matter decreases, the physical structure of soil changes. With less pore space and less of their sponge-like qualities, soils are less efficient at storing water and air. More irrigation is needed. Water leeches through soils, draining away nutrients that no longer have an effective susbstrate on which to cling. With less available oxygen, the growth of soil microbiology slows, and the intricate ecosystem of biological exchanges breaks down."[85]

Tom Philpott, writing for the online magazine *Grist*, shared his personal experience seeing this kind of soil devastation in real life:

"When you look down in an Immokalee tomato field, what you see is sand—there's no evident organic matter in the growing medium (the word "soil" doesn't quite apply here). To prepare for tomato growing, you start by sterilizing the ground with an extremely toxic pesticide—and in the process wipe out any beneficial microbes that might be lingering there. Then you inject the doses of NPK to maximize output, and you're ready to go. (You may need more insecticide sprayings as the season wears on.) More than in any other place I've seen, plants there live on a diet equivalent to sugar water, oat fiber, and vitamin pills. Can there be any real wonder that the resulting tomatoes are so pathetically lacking in flavor? And do people still doubt that they may be less healthful as well?"[86]

Tom Philpott's parting question isn't that far off the mark. A 2007 report analyzed historical records from the U.S. Department of Agriculture and found that many common fruits and vegetables have lower levels of some vitamins and significantly fewer minerals like iron, calcium, and zinc than they did just fifty years ago.[87]

Could it be that this decline in nutrients is the result of a decline in soil health? It doesn't seem all that implausible.

But what about the implications for your personal health? Even if you dismiss the environmental devastation of losing naturally fertile topsoil, there are other reasons to avoid eating pesticide-laden fruits and vegetables.

Produce grown with high-nitrogen fertilizers tends to have more concentrated nitrogen in it. When these extra nitrates enter our highly acidic stomachs, they can be converted into nitrosamines. In a press release announcing a 2009 study released in the *Journal of Alzheimer's Disease*, scientists summed up the documented effects of nitrosamines in the body:

Nitrosamines basically become highly reactive at the cellular level, which then alters gene expression and causes DNA damage. The researchers note that the role of nitrosamines has been well studied, and their role as a carcinogen has been fully documented. The investigators propose that the cellular alterations that occur as a result of nitrosamine exposure are fundamentally similar to those that occur with aging, as well as Alzheimer's, Parkinson's and type 2 diabetes mellitus.[88]

In other words, nitrosamines are a known cancer-causing agent, and they may also contribute to the development of age-related diseases such as Alzheimer's.

The good news about nitrosamines is that if your diet is high in the antioxidant vitamin C, you're not likely to have excess nitrosamine formation. But getting vitamin C from your fruits and vegetables may be harder than you think.

Once a fruit or vegetable is picked, the vitamin content goes down steadily. Cold storage, light, and exposure to air all cause fruits and vegetables to lose vitamins, as does cooking. Potatoes, which are stored for months before making their way to supermarkets and then even longer in your home before you eat them, lose 50% of their vitamin C within two months of harvesting and almost 80% by the time four months have passed. Spinach loses 80% of its vitamins during first two days after harvesting even if it's stored in cool and dark place. And peas? In just a week of storage, they lose 77% of their vitamin C.[89]

The longer the fruit or vegetable is stored, the more vitamins it loses. Because of our modern, insatiable desire to eat all manner of fruits and vegetables out of season—all year 'round—most veggies and fruits are sometimes stored for months at a time before they're finally brought to market.

Not only that, veggies and fruits grown in dead soil have fewer nutrients to start with anyway.

The end result is food that is virtually devoid of vitamins. In fact, one Australian doctor did a series of tests on commercially grown oranges and found that they had no vitamin C at all by the time they were brought to market.[90]

If you want to avoid excess nitrates in your produce, you'll need to buy vegetables and fruits grown without the use of synthetic fertilizers. If you want produce that has the most nutrients in it, you'll need to buy freshly harvested vegetables grown in living, organically rich soil rather than dead, pesticide-laden soil.

So, What Can I Eat?

Overwhelmed yet? Hidden MSG. Processed foods high in genetically modified soy. Corn derivatives that sound like they belong in a chemistry textbook. Refined sweeteners. Industrially raised meats, dairy, and eggs.

Is there anything you *can* eat? Anything at all?

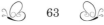

Thankfully, there is. It's called food—real food that's sustainably produced, organically-raised, and locally-grown.

Chapter 4

What to Eat Instead

Navigating the world of grocery stores, natural foods stores, co-ops, farmers markets, and farm stands in an effort to find real, nourishing, non-industrial food can be intimidating. With all the variety and competing health claims, how in the world can you pick the healthiest foods?

After all, we're all real people with budgets, bosses hanging over our shoulders, traffic to battle, marriages to navigate, and friends to encourage. We've got book clubs to frequent, movies to see, dates to go on. In short, we've got a life—a real life that competes for all the time and money you may want to spend in the kitchen cooking or at the store buying food.

How should you prioritize your time and food dollars? If you're opting out of the industrial food system, what else is left? And, how can you afford it?

One of Joel Salatin's favorite quips is, "If you think organic food is expensive, have you priced cancer lately?"

It's a little simplified, but it makes a valid point. In an Oprah appearance on January 27, 2010, food journalist Michael Pollan asked, *"Do you want to pay now for groceries or pay for a doctor later? When I was a kid, we spent 18% of our income on food and 5% on healthcare. Now we spend 9% on food, and 17% on healthcare."*[1] Our country has done an about face. We used to spend a large amount of our income on food, and we didn't get all that sick. Now we buy cheap, industrially produced foods and get chronic diseases that require a lifetime of expensive drugs and medical treatments just to keep us alive. We're not paying for cures, but symptom management.

So, yes, the cost of real food is more expensive. Unlike the corn- and soy-based industrially produced foods, real food is not federally subsidized. Plus, organic and sustainable farmers are often smaller-scale folks who have to operate under expensive, industry-sized yokes. Joel Salatin, when asked why local food was more expensive, shared an anecdote about how his farm entered the mandatory Workman's Comp world when they hired their third employee:

> "Our interns and apprentices, who receive free room and board plus a modest stipend in return for their education, had to be treated

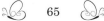

like employees. On our farm, we integrate cattle, pigs, and poultry to such an extent that these different types of animals are in the same area and everyone handles chores for all of them. But in WC land, employees must be segregated between 'Beef and Pork' or 'Poultry.' They can't mix. The risk actuarials are different so they must be separately categorized.

Of course, the risk for cattle and hogs is bigger because they can hurt you, especially in a feedlot or Concentrated Animal Feeding Operation. We have neither. And poultry risk is assessed assuming a confinement fecal particulate fan whirring feed auguring factory house. Ours are in little, squatty pasture schooners, hand-watered, hand-fed, open-air sunshine and dew-speckled pasture.

The real kicker was a delivery driver who takes frozen meat and eggs to the restaurants and home customers. Since we're a farm, we can't have such a delivery driver. The only delivery driver we can have is a live animal hauler—highest risk in the book. If we were a delivery service, we could have a low-risk-delivery driver, but that's impossible with a farm. Farms don't have those kinds of employees.

Bottom line: Our little farm operation is paying more than $10,000 a year for government-mandated Workman's Comp using an assessment system written for Tyson and Cargill. It's absurd. And immoral. Guess who pays that huge cost? The customer. In a thousand different ways, this scenario plays out across the local food movement, arbitrarily and capriciously prejudicing the price. And that, dear friends, is the main reason why local food is more expensive."[2]

Yet, despite its expense, these real foods don't need to break the bank. For more on how to eat real food on a budget, see Appendix B.

Still, you'll want to know how best to prioritize your food dollars. Consider this your guide.

Eat Broth Instead of MSG

The dangers of MSG have been well documented, and not without cause. MSG *really is* dangerous for us. But perhaps even more dangerous than what's in our food is the shocking realization of what's missing. Without bone broths, our diets are sadly out of balance.

Homemade broth is made from the bones of cows, chickens, goats, pigs, and fish. Really, traditional cultures will boil just about any kind of bone to

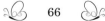

make stock. These homemade broths contain many important minerals in a form your body will easily digest. It's natural to think of calcium first; I do. In fact, broth is the primary way that non-dairy cultures around the world get calcium in their diet. But beyond calcium you've got magnesium, phosphorous, silicon, sulfur, and other trace minerals. Because bone broth also contains broken-down material from tendons and cartilage, it's also rich in other nutrients like chondroitin and glucosamine—now sold as expensive, over-the-counter supplements for arthritis.

Aren't we brilliant? By replacing broth with MSG, we eliminated one of our primary sources of calcium, as well as many vital nutrients for joint health. Then when we suffer from osteoporosis and arthritis, we assume it's just because we're "getting old." We spend a fortune on medicines and artificial supplements trying to undo the damage.

According to Sally Fallon, president of the Weston A. Price foundation, broth plays a significant role in the diet of traditional cultures, "Fish stock, according to traditional lore, helps boys grow up into strong men, makes childbirth easy and cures fatigue. 'Fish broth will cure anything,' is another South American proverb. Broth and soup made with fish heads and carcasses provide iodine and thyroid-strengthening substances."[3] Similarly, Paul Pitchford tells us that bone marrow broth is called "longevity soup" in China.[4] The French people, says Arabella Forge, believe that "A good pot of soup should restore and nourish. In France, the word *restoratif* described soups and stews sold at roadside taverns to weary travelers. They were a source of sustenance for those who were unwell and an antidote to physical exhaustion. The concept of a *restoratif* bowl of soup eventually expanded to describe any place people could stop for a sustaining meal—that is, a restaurant."[5]

People in traditional cultures use broth to create rich, meaty flavors in all kinds of dishes. Of course, soup tops the list. Beef broth makes a good base for many soups and stews from cuisines around the world, such as French Onion Soup, Vietnamese Pho, even plain old Vegetable Soup. Fish broth is paramount in Asian cultures, and chicken broth gets used in old-fashioned American chicken-noodle soup, Irish chicken and dumplings, Tom Kha Ghai in Thailand, and more. Beyond soups, broths can be reduced to make flavorful sauces from around the world—everything from barbecue sauce to curries, Chinese ginger sauce to *au jus*. It can be thickened to create gravies, or used to create a rich flavor when cooking vegetables, risotto, or ratatouille. In the Asian cultures of Japan, Korea, China, and Thailand, mom-and-pop businesses steam up back rooms making broth and sell it on street corners.

Back when we used to butcher animals locally and make use of the whole animal in our cooking, otherwise inedible hooves, bones, knuckles, carcasses, feet, heads, and tough meat went into the stock pot to create a savory, nutrient-dense food that flavored just about everything. Now we've abandoned the tradition of broth making, opting instead for bouillon cubes, dehydrated soup mixes, sauce mixes, and the convenience of fast food.

Today, broth is uncommon in American cuisine. But it's a vibrant part of most traditional cultures, particularly those that eat less meat than we do. That's because the gelatin in broth also helps the body assimilate protein, so you can stretch meat further when you serve it in a meal with a properly made, nutrient-dense bone broth. Again, Sally Fallon elaborates:

> "When broth is cooled, it congeals due to the presence of gelatin. The use of gelatin as a therapeutic agent goes back to the ancient Chinese…. Although gelatin is not a complete protein, containing only the amino acids arginine and glycine in large amounts, it acts as a protein sparer, helping the poor stretch a few morsels of meat into a complete meal. During the siege of Paris, when vegetables and meat were scarce, a doctor named Guerard put his patients on gelatin bouillon with some added fat and they survived in good health."[6]

Gelatin is also loaded with two necessary amino acids: proline and glycine. Maybe you've heard of them? They're two integral parts of your body's connective tissue. Without proline and glycine, your body would literally fall apart. They're in *everything*. The cartilage that forms your joints? Check. The collagen that keeps wrinkles at bay? Check. The cellular structure that acts as a scaffold for the cells in your muscles, arteries, and organs? Check. We need these two amino acids to heal open wounds as well as inflammation. They can ease digestion, calm your mood, improve your memory, and clear up blocked arteries and blood vessels.[7]

Making homemade broth isn't all that difficult, and I even share a recipe for it in the second half of this book. So, you don't have an excuse! Ditch the MSG and opt for broth instead.

Eat Traditional Fats & Oils

What kinds of fats and oils did traditional cultures rely on before modern, seed-based cooking oils were invented?

Only a handful of plants readily gave edible oils to us without requiring industrial solvents or complex extraction techniques: coconuts, palm trees, olives, avocados, and oily nuts like the macadamia. Animals, on the other hand, were flush with fat. The fat could easily be collected, cooked down and purified into tallow, lard, and schmaltz. Even dairy animals offered up fatty cream which could be churned into butter or clarified to make ghee.

In recent years, many of these ancient fats and oils have been demonized because they're swimming with saturated fat. You shouldn't let that scare you. For more on why saturated fat isn't inherently dangerous, read Chapter 7.

I like to think about these fats and oils in terms of how to use them in the kitchen, dividing them up according to whether or not I'll cook with them or simply use them as a condiment.

Fats & Oils for Cooking

Fat or Oil	Safe Cooking Temperatures
Butter from grass-fed cows	Lower than 350°F
Coconut Oil or Palm Kernel Oil, preferably unrefined and low-temperature extracted	Lower than 350°F, does well in baked goods
Lard from foraged pigs	Lower than 370°F, good replacement for vegetable shortening
Schmaltz from pastured poultry	Lower than 375°F
Macadamia Oil, cold-pressed	Lower than 410°F, excellent for stir-fries
Red Palm Oil, unrefined	Lower than 410°F, good for popcorn
Tallow from grass-fed cows	Lower than 420°F, great for French fries
Ghee from grass-fed cows	Lower than 425°F
Avocado Oil, cold-pressed, UV-protected	Lower than 520°F

When using fats to cook, there are a couple of things to note. The first is that any animal fats should be sourced from grass-fed, wild, or pastured animals. This will ensure that the animal ate a traditional diet and itself has

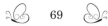

a traditional balance of fats. For example, the omega-6 to omega-3 ratio for products from an industrialized cow is 21:1. For a grass-fed and finished cow, it can be as low as 1:1 and is generally no higher than 4:1. The second thing to note is to avoid cooking fats past their smoke point.

When a fat is exposed to high enough temperatures, it starts to smoke, starting the process of oxidization. Most scientific research agrees that oxidized fats lead to inflammation of the arteries—the underlying cause of heart disease. Oxidization has also been linked to increasing risks of cancer, presumably because of the extra free radicals racing around our bodies.

Fats & Oils for Condiments

The next table features fats and oils that make good condiments (in other words, they're good served cool or warm).

Fat or Oil	Uses
Olive Oil, cold-pressed, UV-protected	Salad dressings, warmed or gently-cooked foods, mayonnaise
Sesame Oil, cold-pressed, in small quantities because of the high concentration of PUFAs	Salad dressings, dips, Asian dishes
Avocado Oil, cold-pressed, UV-protected	Salad dressings, dips
Macadamia Oil, cold-pressed	Salad dressings, mayonnaise
Coconut Oil, unrefined, low-temperature extracted	Smoothies, mayonnaise, raw desserts
Butter from grass-fed cows	Hollandaise sauce, over sautéed vegetables
Sour Cream, full-fat, with live, active cultures	Dips, stirred into cooling soups & stews, on tacos!
Yogurt, full-fat, with live, active cultures	Dips, salad dressings, stirred into cooling dishes

When using fats as condiments, we're talking about using them in salad dressings or spreads, to drizzle over steamed vegetables, to stir into cooling soups or stews, and the like. The most important things to note for these fats is that they're as natural and as traditionally made as possible, and that they're properly stored. For most of the oils, you need to make sure they were cold-pressed rather than extracted via high-temperature or high-pressure

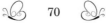

processing, and that they were extracted without the use of chemical solvents. For the fats with living cultures of bacteria (like sour cream and yogurt), you'll want to make sure you don't heat them above 118° F. Otherwise, you kill the bacteria cultures and remove the probiotic benefit of the food.

Eat Wild- and Pasture-Fed-Animal Foods

Before factory farming took hold fifty years ago, cattle were raised on family ranches and farms. The process was a little wild and quite natural. Baby calves were born in the spring and spent months with their mothers nursing and munching on lush spring grasses. The calves matured at a natural pace, taking nearly three years to reach market weight. They were then slaughtered, aged in a cool place for a couple weeks to improve tenderness and flavor, and shipped to your local meat market where your butcher would divide the meat up into individual cuts at your request.

Unlike the supermarket meat of today, "This meat was free of antibiotics, added hormones, feed additives, flavor enhancers, age-delaying gases and saltwater solutions. Mad cow disease and the deadliest strain of E. coli—0157:H7—did not exist. People dined on rare steaks and steak tartare (raw ground beef) with little fear."[8]

If you want to return to the pre-factory farming model of eating meat, the best way to do it is by eating wild animals or pasture-raised livestock. Eating wild animals needs little explanation. You or someone you know grabs a rifle, shotgun, or fishing equipment and heads into the great outdoors to hunt, trap, or catch something unsullied by industry to eat.

But why the emphasis on pasture-fed livestock? And why is it so much better than what you can eat within the factory farmed, industrial model?

Three letters: CLA.

What is CLA? It's Conjugated Linoleic Acid, and it's only found in the fat of grazing ruminants like cattle and sheep. And, because a pasture-raised hen eats lots of green grass, her eggs are another great source of CLA.

Scientific research is proving time and again that this stuff:

- Combats cancer[9 10 11 12 13 14 15 16 17 18 19 20]
- Fights clogged arteries [21 22]
- Reduces body fat[23]
- Ameliorates digestive inflammation due to IBS, Chron's disease[24 25]

Plus, while industrially raised, corn-fed meats and dairy have an omega-6 to omega-3 ratio hovering around 20:1, an entirely grass-fed cow has a much more ideal ratio of 1:1.

Apart from having an appealing fat profile, animals raised on pasture also have a beneficial impact on the earth. For example, rotating cattle through pastures by allowing them to intensively graze on young, shooting grass builds an inch of fertile top soil every year![26] That's because grass grows down as well as up. When a cow walks by and chews off the top of the grass, the plant sheds an equal amount of roots, building the soil. It takes approximately 500 years for nature alone to produce an inch of topsoil, but an intensively grazed field can build it in relatively no time.

In the current industrial model of farming, we grow a sea of corn in Iowa to feed cattle in California or Texas. Rather than raising the cattle in a self-contained system, we raise them in a feedlot that requires inputs of food, fuel, and water while simultaneously polluting the air and nearby waterways. Because of these current methods, we *lose an inch of topsoil every twenty-eight years*. In the last hundred years, we've lost more than a third of our topsoil![27] We cannot continue to grow a giant sea of corn to feed our livestock for the next hundred years. Imagine the dustbowl of the 1930s that swept away entire towns and cities, but on a nationwide scale. We have to return our animals to the land so that they can nourish it and build it while also drawing sustenance from it.

Cows not only add to the soil simply by being ruminants, they also add to the fertility of the soil and fields with their poop. Poop is perhaps the most prolific source of organic matter we have, and yet all we do in a factory farm is throw it away. A cow can shed around fifty pounds of poop per day. In a factory farm, the poop sits on the ground, dries out, and washes away into a toxic manure lagoon near the feedlot. In the meantime, crop farmers will spend $15,000 or more on fertilizer in a year.

Are you finally seeing the conundrum? Crop farmers who grow monoculture crops like corn, soy, or rapeseed have to buy fertilizer to replace the fertility they lost when they moved cattle and other animals off their farms.

An integrated farm with a variety of animals and crops can be vastly more productive and have far fewer inputs; plus, it's actually sustainable for the long haul.

So, now that you know that pasture-based animal husbandry is better—for the animals, for the food they produce, and for the environment—I think it's time we get down to the nitty-gritty. How can you prioritize your food purchases?

For Meat

BEST CHOICE: The meat from grass-fed/pastured/foraged/wild animals. This can often be expensive if you're buying it by the cut at a natural foods store, so I cannot stress highly enough the need to get your hands on a large freezer and buy in bulk directly from farmers. With your grocery savings alone, you'll probably pay for that freezer in less than a year or two. Economize even more by hunting wild game and picking up specially discounted meats at your local farmer's market. Or, if you have land, consider raising your own animals to feed your family and a few neighbors.

SECOND CHOICE: Buy meat that is third-party certified for farming practices (some decent certifications include the USDA Certified Organic label, the Animal Welfare Approved label, and the Certified Humane label). Or, in the very least, buy those that specifically claim to be "raised without the use of antibiotics or hormones." I say this because one very deceptive practice that boils my blood every time I think about it is the labeling of meat, such as chicken, as "naturally raised," "hormone-free," or "antibiotic-free" with a tiny little asterisk after the claim. First of all, "naturally raised" is not a regulated term and doesn't *necessarily* mean anything. Furthermore, that little asterisk? If you take the time to hunt down the modifying language on the company's website or literature, you'll almost always find out that they simply mean they don't use hormones or antibiotics in the *processing* of the animal.

This has nothing to do with how the animal was raised, and everything to do with how it was cut up and packaged. In other words, it's a completely empty claim. Who uses antibiotics or hormones when packaging meat? Don't be deceived! You're paying a premium for something not substantially different than any other industrialized meat.

So, by sticking to certified meat or meat that specifically claims to be "raised without the use of antibiotics or hormones," you are at least guaranteeing that these potentially harmful and toxic substances aren't in the fat, marrow, or meat of the animal you're eating.

THIRD CHOICE: Buy meats that are additive and preservative free. Avoid MSG, nitrates & nitrites, etc. by carefully reading labels. Sometimes even these labels can be deceptive, particularly in the case of lunchmeats and sausages. (For this reason, my family doesn't buy deli or lunchmeat any more. Instead, we'll make our own using roasts. Or, we sometimes slice up liverwurst, braunschweiger, or other organ meat sausages from grass-fed animals).

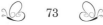

For Dairy

Given my lengthy description of everything wrong with industrially produced milk in the last chapter, you may be surprised to know that I actually believe milk can be a healthy food choice. The key here is to stick to milk choices that are traditional—the kind your ancestors have been drinking and turning into cultured foods like yogurt, cheese, kefir, buttermilk, and sour cream for thousands of years.

BEST CHOICE: Raw, non-homogenized whole milk and raw cheeses from grass-fed cows producing milk high in A2 beta casein and relatively low in A1 beta casein—that means milk from Jerseys, Guernseys, and other traditional cattle breeds rather than newer Holsteins. Raw, non-homogenized goat's milk, sheep's milk, and yak's milk only contains A2 beta casein, so you could make a great argument for giving raw goat's milk preference over raw cow's milk if you can find it.

SECOND CHOICE: Raw, non-homogenized whole milk and raw cheeses from other grass-fed cows. This is almost identical to the first and best choice, and is only rated slightly lower in my opinion because it comes from newer cattle breeds rather than the more traditional varieties.

THIRD CHOICE: Pasteurized (but not ultra high temperature pasteurized), non-homogenized whole milk and cheeses from grass-fed cows. Some states have laws requiring farmers to pasteurize their milk if they're selling it. Despite the pasteurization, it is still worth paying the premium to get milk that is from grass-fed cows and hasn't been homogenized.

FOURTH CHOICE: Pasteurized, homogenized whole milk from grass-fed cows. Because this milk has been homogenized, it rates slightly lower than the non-homogenized milk above. Included in this last acceptable (but far from ideal) category are pasteurized cheeses from milk that comes from cows raised without growth hormones or antibiotics. Because the cheese has been naturally cultured with enzymes and bacteria, it makes it worth eating despite the fact that it hasn't come from entirely grass-fed cows.

If you can't get your hands on milk from grass-fed cows at all, I wouldn't bother drinking it. There'd be almost nothing distinguishing it from the industrial milk in your supermarket. Instead, I'd stick to a homemade milk substitute like a coconut milk tonic or a homemade almond milk.

For Eggs

So, faced with the myriad of meaningless supermarket egg labels, how can you choose the most nourishing, healthy eggs for your family?

BEST CHOICE: Pastured eggs from a local farmer. Chickens live their entire lives outdoors, in the pasture, picking through cow dung, eating bugs and grass, basking in the sun. Their feed may or may not be supplemented with anything other than what God and Nature provide in the field. If it is supplemented, a non-soy feed is best. Pick these up at your local farmer's markets, or use Craigslist or another local ad service to find someone raising hens who would like to part with excess eggs.

Remember, when compared to the USDA's nutrient data for conventional eggs coming from chickens confined in factory farms, the eggs of pastured hens usually contain:[28]

- 1/3 less cholesterol
- 1/4 less saturated fat
- 2/3 more vitamin A
- 2 times more omega-3 fatty acids
- 3 times more vitamin E
- 7 times more beta-carotene
- 4 to 6 times more vitamin D

SECOND CHOICE: At the supermarket, choose the eggs with the most omega-3s and DHAs available. Those are the nutrients most commonly lacking in the eggs from "battery hens," and some companies have specially formulated their chicken feed in an attempt to make up for the hen's abnormal and unnatural living conditions. Still produced in heinous factory farm situations, these eggs are likely to come from hens routinely fed low-level antibiotics. But, at least these eggs *attempt* to make up for the nutrient deficiencies inherent in the system.

THIRD CHOICE: Organic eggs. I often waver between switching this choice with the one above, and I've decided that it's a matter of personal choice for each of us. Although they may not be nutritionally superior to your average "battery hen" eggs, you at least know these eggs came from hens raised without the use of antibiotics and that the hens were fed organic feed. According to the Cornucopia Institute, they are still likely to be

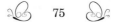

produced in factory farm situations.[29] But there are some organic producers out there who don't fit the industry mold, and you should give yourself the freedom to support them.

For Seafood

Without a doubt, our oceans are polluted and over-fished. Our streams are thoroughly saturated with mercury—a deadly poison.[30] This has led many to throw up their hands in despair and swear off seafood altogether.

That's not a good choice.

Seafood is an incredibly nutrient-dense food—arguably the best source for fat-soluble vitamins A & D, omega-3 fatty acids, and more. According to the research of Dr. Weston A. Price, traditional people groups around the world prized seafood above every other food and went to great lengths to obtain it, regardless of their location.

That was certainly true on Viti Levu, one of the larger islands that make up the Fiji Island group. As he recounts in *Nutrition and Physical Degeneration,* Dr. Price visited there and learned that the natives considered seafood so essential that the hill tribes and the coast tribes would exchange plant foods from the mountain areas for seafood from the coast. Even more remarkable, says Price, is that fact that the tribal members entrusted with carrying these foods to the storehouses of the other tribes were "never molested, not even during active warfare."[31]

Did you catch that? Even in times of war with coastal tribes, when their normal access routes would be cut off, inland tribes still sought out seafood. Perhaps more telling is that the coastal tribes still freely traded with them.

But, you say, what about mercury in fish? Surely that wasn't such a problem back in Dr. Price's day? Isn't that a good enough reason to stop eating it?

Not according to Sally Fallon Morell, president of the Weston A. Price Foundation. She has said that her research has indicated that if you have good gut flora, you are protected from the mercury in fish![32] So, if you are eating a diet rich in lacto-fermented foods and/or taking a good probiotic supplement, the mercury content of fish is less of an issue. Also, a study done on rats found that those with normal gut flora had no problem eliminating a mercury toxin from their system, while those with damaged gut flora (induced by a course of antibiotics) developed symptoms of mercury toxicity.[33]

So, what are the healthiest seafoods you can buy?

BEST CHOICE: Mollusks are the most nutrient-dense of all seafoods. Oysters, clams, mussels, scallops, octopus, and squid are the most commonly available mollusks in your grocery store. And these days, many of these foods are farmed using such sustainable practices that the farmed versions are actually better for you and the environment than their wild-caught counterparts thanks to the heavy pollution and over-fishing of the wild. Depending on where you live, you can find these fresh, frozen, or canned.

SECOND CHOICE: Other shellfish such as lobster, crayfish, shrimp, and crabs are also significantly more nutrient-dense than fish, though less so than mollusks. As with mollusks, many of the farmed versions of these seafoods are now so sustainably farmed that they exceed their wild counterparts in sustainability & healthfulness. Also included in this second list are fish roe (eggs), available fresh or jarred. They're an essential part of most native fertility diets—and for good reason!

THIRD CHOICE: Fish—any fish. Oily fish are among the most nutrient-dense, but also among the ones that warrant the most caution with regard to sustainability and toxicity. Sticking to small, oily fish like sardines and anchovies can virtually eliminate any risk of toxicity. In general, wild-caught carnivorous fish are significantly more nutrient-dense than their farmed counterparts, mostly because of the unnatural diets fed to the farmed fish. According to Nina Planck, if the fish are herbivorous (like tilapia), then it's easy to feed them their natural diet, although few aquatic farms do.[34]

But, as always, the choice between wild and farmed fish needs to be made on an individual case-by-case basis. For example, there are only a handful of authentically sustainable tilapia farms in the world that prioritize feeding the fish their natural diet and developing natural ecosystems. So, for most of us, sticking to wild-caught, sustainably harvested fish is best.

So, how do you balance the nutrient-density of these foods against their sustainability and toxicity?

Easy.

The folks at the Monterey Bay Aquarium have put together the most comprehensive database of seafood, farming and harvesting practices, and toxicity levels available today. And, they've conveniently condensed all this information into a handy pocket shopping guide, which is broken down according to region. The pocket guides are divided into three categories: Best Choices, Good Alternatives, and Avoid. I personally shop from this guide for my region, choosing mollusks, shellfish, and fish (in that order) according to what's best and what's on sale. You can download the guide online at: www.montereybayaquarium.org/cr/cr_seafoodwatch/download.aspx

Eat Natural Sweeteners

On a biological level, sugar is still sugar. You'll want to limit your intake of it, regardless of the form it comes in.

But what do you do when it's your husband's birthday and you want to indulge in a dessert? Or you get a promotion and want to celebrate? What do you do when it's time to sit down to a breakfast of sourdough waffles?

Thank goodness for natural sweeteners.

This may seem obvious, but as more and more dubious products hit the market claiming to be "natural" sweeteners, I think it's time to set the record straight. A natural sweetener is one that a person could reasonably expect to grow, harvest, and process themselves without the use of added chemicals, enzymes, or expensive machinery. It's a traditional sweetener, used in moderation for centuries, if not longer.

So, let's do a quick exercise.

I'm going to name some sweeteners that claim to be "natural," and I want you to tell me if they're actually natural or not.

Let's start with some easy ones. Honey? Yes, I could imagine a scenario where I raised honeybees. I don't choose to do that right now, but it's possible. Maple Syrup? Again, yes. I don't live in Vermont, and I don't have maple trees to tap. But if I did, I could. And then I could boil it down to make syrup. Thousands of people do just this every year.

Now, let's tackle some more complicated ones. How about Sorghum Syrup? Again, this is a crop that I could grow, but don't. Theoretically, I could press the sorghum cane to get juice that I could then simmer until it turns into syrup. It'd be a lot of work, but I could do it—all with pre-industrial technology. So, yes, it's a natural sweetener. How about Sucanat? This is a naturally evaporated juice from the sugar cane, but you evaporated it until crystals form rather than a syrup. I definitely don't live in the Caribbean, and I don't grow sugar cane. But I *could* live there, and if I did, I could work with other farm laborers to create this sweetener. What about Turbinado Sugar? Here's where it gets tricky. They like to call this "evaporated cane juice" to make it sound natural, but really it's just refined sugar that's had a smidgeon of molasses added back into it to give it a golden hue. So, no, it's not natural.

What about sugar alcohols like xylitol and erythritol? Well, since these are isolated nutrients that require laboratories to produce, I think it's safe to say that these aren't natural sweeteners. The same thing is true of highly processed takes on stevia like Truvia and PureVia.

Are you starting to get the idea? While I don't actually grow or process any of these natural sweeteners myself, I know *how* it's done and know that I could do it myself. The point here isn't that I actually make all my own natural sweeteners, just that I could (given the right circumstances).

Every region of the world has a native sweetener. I suggest you find out what's normal for your area, and go eat it!

So, what sweeteners do I, personally, eat? In my own home, we try to choose natural sweeteners that are easily available. If a natural sweetener isn't listed here, it's not necessarily because I think it's not natural. It's just that it's not casually available to me locally within my budget.

STEVIA

Stevia is an herb that tastes sweet on the tongue without any actual sugar molecules to send your metabolism into a tailspin. As such, it's awfully nice to use when you're trying to reduce sugar intake or go low-carb. The white, powdered versions of Stevia out there are highly refined mysteries and therefore suspect. I'm not saying it's impossible to make a white, powdered version of Stevia in my own kitchen, but I just don't know how I'd do it. And unfortunately for most of the companies selling the stuff, they're not willing to disclose how they do it either. So, for now, I'll assume it's some kind of weird, chemically enhanced refining process and stay away from the stuff.

That said, the green-leaf stevia is a plant that I grow on my own patio. It is as local as it comes. I've used it for the following:

- Adding fresh or dried leaves to tealeaves or other herbal teas before brewing in order to add a natural sweetness without the use of sugar.

- Making a liquid stevia extract using vodka, which I then use to do things like make homemade chocolate milk for my kids or sweeten already brewed or cold beverages.

COCONUT PALM SUGAR

Almost every grocery store near me carries this on the sugar aisle, right next to the turbinado and so-called "raw" sugars that really aren't. Coconut sugar is made by evaporating the sap from the coconut tree. In the Philippines and Indonesia, it is common to turn older, taller, less-productive coconut trees into "sap trees"—trees dedicated entirely to sap production rather than growing coconuts. These trees are usually around homes and public

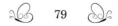

parks where they're valued for the shade they provide. The added advantage of not having falling coconuts (which kill more people there than lightning strikes!) also tends to mean that yards and parks are safer for families.[35] I use this sugar in baked goods or other recipes that call for granulated sugar. I can substitute it fairly well for table sugar without it dramatically altering the final consistency or flavor of the recipe. Although it is still sugar and still bad for you, at least it's unrefined and has the naturally occurring trace minerals present.

SUCANAT & MUSCOVADO

My ability to get my hands on these sweeteners is rather hit and miss. But when I can get them, I do. Because they are unrefined, evaporated juice from the sugar cane, they have a rich molasses flavor and make excellent substitutes for recipes that call for brown sugar.

RAW HONEY

A little old lady sells the most amazing honey at my weekly farmer's market. She keeps bees in her yard, and has been selling honey at my town's farmer's market for almost her entire life. I stir this into hot beverages, use it to sweeten dips or dressings, and use it to make my favorite ice cream. I very rarely substitute honey for granulated sugar in recipes as it has a strong (and different!) flavor as well as a different consistency.

MAPLE SYRUP

This occasionally gets used to top our grain-free pancakes. I'm sure there are other uses for it, but that's all this sweetener does in our house.

SORGHUM SYRUP

This, too, occasionally gets used to top our pancakes. Sorghum syrup is a traditional natural sweetener used in the American deep South, but originally hails from Africa. I use it over almond-flour biscuits and in my pecan pie as a replacement for corn syrup.

Eat Properly Prepared Grains

You'd think it'd be simple. Eating grains is as old as… well, agriculture. But within the last century the industrialized grains we eat have become quite perverted. Refined flours have weaseled their way into just about every baked good: breads, cereals, crackers, desserts, you name it.

When I was a kid, you couldn't get me to eat white bread. My mother had raised us on whole wheat bread—at least that's what the label said it was. We'd use the soft, but darker bread to make sandwiches. Every morning for many years I'd pack my own lunch. A brown paper bag. A whole wheat ham and cheese sandwich with mayo. A bag of Doritos. A Little Debbie snack cake. An apple. Sometimes I'd be daring and pack a banana.

At some point, that little girl grew into a young woman, gained some independence, and started reading ingredient labels. Turns out, my "whole wheat" bread wasn't whole wheat at all. The first—and therefore primary—ingredient on the label was unbleached wheat flour, not whole wheat flour. It said it right there in black and white; I saw my illusions crumbling. The difference between my Nature's Made Honey Wheat sandwich bread and Iron Kids bread? A few tablespoons of whole-wheat flour, but not enough to make any significant difference health wise.

Since then, I've learned that even whole-grains—the so-called "healthy" alternative—are dangerously devoid of nutrients thanks to our modern methods of grain preparation.

We all know that refined grains are "bad" for us. In the refining process, the bran and germ are removed from the whole-grain, hence removing the fiber and most of the vitamins and minerals. Then the grains are further processed via mixing, bleaching, and brominating.

When poor people with limited diets switched to eating these refined and improperly prepared grains, they began suffering from devastating vitamin and mineral deficiencies—sometimes in epidemic proportions.

Perhaps the two most famous examples of this were in Asia and in the American deep South. In Asia, as more and more of the population began eating polished white rice, a terrifying outbreak swept the continent. A new disease called beriberi infected thousands upon thousands of people. In their quest to determine the cause of the disease, researchers discovered vitamins—a heretofore unknown component of our food. In this case, they stumbled upon the B-complex vitamins inherent in brown rice, which were being removed with the bran when polishing the rice. By enriching polished

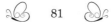

rice with synthetic B vitamins, the epidemic was stopped in its tracks.[36] Likewise, the American South faced an outbreak of pellagra when subsistence farmers facing an economic downturn tried to survive on a corn-based diet. In 1916, more than 100,000 southerners came down with the disease. Unlike the American natives, who also ate a corn-based diet, these southerners didn't soak their corn overnight in the mineral lime. The soaking process—called nixtamalization—breaks down the antinutrients present in corn and increases the availability of vitamins, in this case niacin.[37] When pellagra was finally linked to a vitamin deficiency, they recommended that people supplement their diet with a few tablespoons of brewer's yeast (another rich source of B vitamins) to curtail the epidemic.

When we learned that milled and improperly prepared grains could wreak such havoc among the poorest among us, we began "enriching" the refined grains with synthetic vitamins and minerals.

In nature, nutrients don't appear in isolation. Yet all of these synthetic vitamins are created in isolation, in laboratories. These vitamin isolates can have unintended consequences. In 1995, researchers wanted to track the role of vitamin A in pregnant women. Rather than enhancing the participant's diets with foods naturally high in vitamin A, the scientists prescribed a simple vitamin A supplement. The results were utterly shocking and tragic, causing the researchers to immediately stop the study and publish their findings. What happened? The miscarriage rate in women who supplemented with synthetic vitamin A went up 400%.[38]

If possible, you should avoid taking these synthetic vitamins and minerals and stick to correcting any nutritional deficiencies with food.

Even if I supposed that these vitamin isolates were substantially equivalent to naturally occurring vitamins and minerals, the vitamin and mineral content artificially added back into enriched flours still does not measure up to the amount inherent in whole-grains.

Without question, whole-grains are nutritionally superior to refined grains. But what happens to these whole-grains when we mill them at high temperatures, divvy them up into bran, germ, and starch, extrude them into playful breakfast cereal shapes, or simply prepare them without traditional grain preparation techniques?

Sure, our ancestors included whole-grains as a staple in their diet. But did they really make use of them like we do today?

Let's take a quick tour of traditional cultures around the world and see how they prepare and eat grains.

- **India**—Rice and lentils are fermented for at least two days before they are prepared as *idli* and *dosas* or *uttapam*.

- **Ethiopia**—Teff is fermented for three days and used to prepare a tangy flatbread called *injera*.

- **Africa**—Corn, sorghum, or millet is soaked in water for three days, then wet milled and fermented for several more days before being cooked into a porridge or shaped into dough balls called *ogi*.

- **Mexico**—Corn is soaked in a warm water and mineral lime solution for days before being wet milled into a corn flour that's used to make *tortillas*, *gorditas*, and other flat bread.

- **Middle East**—Cracked wheat is fermented in yogurt, then dried and ground into a flour called *kishk*, which is then used as the base for soups and gravies.

- **South America**—Corn is soaked in a warm water and mineral lime solution for at least one day, then wet milled into a sticky dough, formed into balls, and wrapped with banana leaves. These balls are left alone to ferment for an additional two weeks before the finished *pozol* is ready to eat.

- **Europe**—Dried wheat or rye is ground into flour that's then mixed with water and a sourdough starter (a culture of bacteria and wild yeast that is carefully maintained by the bread maker). This new mixture ferments for at least another 8 hours before forming dough that's shaped into loaves and then baked, making *sourdough bread*. Oats or other grains were soaked overnight, sometimes as long as several days in water or soured milk before they were cooked and served as *porridge*.

- **Asia**—Every Asian culture traditionally fermented their rice. Sometimes it's a simple overnight soaking before cooking rice for meals. Other times it's a complicated multi-day wild fermentation with various mixtures of mold, bacteria, and yeast to produce bases like *Red Yeast Rice* in China, *Tape Katan* in Indonesia, or *Koji* in Japan.

What do all of these traditional methods have in common? The grain is always prepared by at least one, if not a combination of these methods:

- **Sprouting**—This is when the whole-grain kernel is sprouted. You can eat it as is, or you can dry it again before grinding it into flour.

- **Soaking**—This is when the already milled whole-grain flour is soaked in an acidic medium like buttermilk, whey, yogurt, lemon juice, or vinegar before being cooked.

- **Fermenting**—This is when the grain is naturally fermented with wild bacteria or yeast, as is the case with all sourdough breads.

Almost all of these methods of grain preparation have been abandoned by us in our haste and love of convenience. We can't blame our parents or our grandparent's generation for falling in love with the easier food preparation industry brought us. Modern science revolutionized our lives, reduced the amount of time and energy it took us to perform tasks, and gave us more time to do the things we really enjoyed. It also revolutionized our food, dramatically reducing the time we spent in the kitchen preparing wholesome meals.

But this convenience came at a cost. We lost many wonderful food traditions as Grandmas raved about frozen pizzas and stopped cooking from scratch. We stopped eating meals together around a table, instead opting for fast food on the go. And the traditional food preparation techniques that had nourished us for thousands of years fell victim to the efficiency of industrialization.

Now, instead of capturing wild yeast from the air through the long process of sourdough fermentation, we had quick rising baker's yeast. And instead of soaking our whole-grain flour in buttermilk overnight to produce wonderfully light and fluffy buttermilk pancakes in the morning, we could use a baking mix containing white flour and chemical leavening agents to achieve the same effect.

So what? How does this affect the food's nutrition?

Grains are essentially the seeds of domesticated grasses. Seeds are meant to do one thing: propagate their species. They are built with multiple layers of protection in order to pass through the digestive systems of animals unharmed so that they can grow in a new place where the animals deposited them. Anyone who's ever raised chickens and fed them kitchen scraps can attest to this. How many of us have had "volunteer" vegetables like squash or tomatoes spring up where our chickens have pooped? Compared to your average chicken, we have teeth and a fairly acidic digestive tract, so we do a better job at breaking down the seeds and grains.

But grains are still hard on our digestive systems, and we don't digest any grain completely. Undigested particles of grain called lectins get stuck in the microvilli of our intestinal walls, building up with time, and ultimately

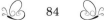

undermining our ability to properly digest other foods because of this interference.[39] If the interference becomes extreme, a host of intestinal and auto-immune disorders can result, including leaky-gut syndrome, gluten intolerance, celiac disease, and irritable-bowel syndrome.[40]

On top of all this, we have to battle phytic acid—the enzyme inhibitor present in grains that locks up all the minerals and vitamins until the seed is ready to germinate. When that phytic acid gets loose in our own guts, it binds with the vitamins and minerals present and keeps us from absorbing them.[41] This can lead to a host of systemic problems, most notably dental decay.[42]

It turns out that traditional grain preparation techniques solved these problems!

Soaking whole-grain flour in an acidic medium overnight neutralizes the phytic acid by activating phytase[43]—an enzyme present in the grain which breaks down the phytic acid, rendering the grain easier for us to digest.

Fermenting whole-grain flour also neutralizes the phytic acid and does an even more thorough job breaking the grain down[44] [45]—to the point that many who suffer from gluten intolerance have no trouble eating traditionally prepared sourdough bread!

And sprouting grains not only neutralizes the phytic acid,[46] but also radically increases the nutrients present. This is because the grain has essentially been turned into a vegetable. When comparing sprouted wheat with unsprouted wheat on a calorie-per-calorie basis, the sprouted wheat contains:[47]

- four times the amount of niacin
- nearly twice the amount of vitamin B6 and folate
- five times the amount of vitamin C
- significantly more protein and fewer starches and sugars

If you're going to eat grains, you should really make sure they are traditionally prepared. For many recipes, this consists of making a few minor and easy adaptations. For example, you can soak your rolled oats overnight in yogurt before adding water and cooking in the morning. This is how traditional cultures have always prepared their porridge, and it only takes a few extra minutes in addition to a little planning to eat this instead of quick cooking instant oatmeal. You can also do this with your breakfast quick breads like pancakes and biscuits simply by soaking the whole-wheat flour in buttermilk overnight before adding the rest of the recipe's ingredients and cooking in the morning.

Perhaps the easiest way to adapt to eating healthier grains is to simply substitute sprouted-grain flour for your typical whole-grain flour. If you have a grain grinder, you can sprout the grain yourself, dry it, and grind it into fresh flour. (This is what I do whenever I occasionally eat grains.) Or, if you don't have a grinder, you can buy sprouted grain flour. Although sometimes hard to find locally, sprouted-grain flour is easy to find and purchase online.

Chapter 5

Taking Care of the Gut

Hippocrates—the ancient Greek father of medicine—once said that "all diseases begin in the gut." Although his understanding of medicine was primitive compared to today, modern research has revealed he wasn't too far off the mark. Our gut is a primary line of defense in our immune system. But, perhaps more revealing is what we're learning about how our gut affects our primary nervous system—altering our moods, keeping our mental acuity sharp, affecting our memory, and more.

Sandra Blakeslee, a science journalist for *The New York Times* once led an article on gut health with the following questions:

"Ever wonder why people get 'butterflies' in the stomach before going on stage? Or why an impending job interview can cause an attack of intestinal cramps? And why antidepressants targeted for the brain cause nausea or abdominal upset in millions of people who take such drugs?

The reason for these common experiences, scientists say, is that the body has two brains—the familiar one encased in the skull and a lesser-known but vitally important one found in the human gut. Like Siamese twins, the two brains are interconnected; when one gets upset, the other does, too."[1]

Her article quotes Dr. Michael Gershon, a professor of anatomy and cell biology at Columbia-Presbyterian Medical Center in New York. The good doctor happily applies a label to your gut that you may have never considered. He calls it your "second brain."

It turns out your gut has more than 100 million neurons—more nerves than your spinal column has. We call it the "enteric nervous system" as opposed to the "central nervous system" comprised of your brain and spinal column. In almost every way, your gut's nervous system acts like your brain does. Your brain has glial cells that nourish neurons? So does your gut. Your brain has mast cells involved in immune responses? So does your gut. Your brain has a "blood brain barrier" that keeps harmful substances away from important nerves? So does your gut. Your brain has sensors to help regulate its functioning? So does your gut. Your brain creates neurotransmitters to help relay information and regulate moods? So does your gut. In fact, more than 80% of your body's serotonin, the so-called "happy" neurotransmitter that helps keep your mood serene is made in your gut. Furthermore, none of your gut's neural pathways are simple. They are just as integrated and complex as the circuits in your brain.[2]

These two nervous systems—your central nervous system and your enteric nervous system—are deeply connected. Early in the development of the human embryo, a collection of tissue called the 'neural crest' appears and divides. One part turns into the central nervous system, and the other becomes the enteric nervous system. Later on in fetal development, these two unique nervous systems link through a neural cable called the vagus nerve, a nerve that begins in your brain and ends in your abdomen. As the longest nerve in the human body, it forms a brain-gut connection that helps explain how and why the health of your gut is so integral to the health of your brain.

So what makes a healthy gut?

In their article "The Long Hollow Tube," Sally Fallon and Mary Enig, Ph.D. describe the gut this way:

"The digestive system is far more than a collection of pipes, wiring and membranes. It is actually an ecosystem, populated by billions of organisms that produce substances necessary for digestion to occur—enzymes, vitamins and beneficial acids (especially lactic acid).... When the intestinal ecosystem is healthy, beneficial bacteria keep yeasts and other fermentation microorganisms at bay in this part of the digestive tract. An imbalance of microorganisms, called *dysbiosis*, results in overgrowth of fungus and other pathogens, resulting in numerous digestive disorders.... Like all ecosystems, the delicate balance of the digestive tract can be altered by various toxins including antibiotics and other drugs, chemicals like chlorine and fluoride in our water, food additives and preservatives, stimulants like coffee, and an overabundance of difficult-to-digest foods like improperly prepared whole grains."[3]

When the balance of microorganisms in your gut is out of balance and the "bad bacteria" proliferate, these bad bacteria produce toxins that can weaken your immune response. They also interfere with the proper absorption of nutrients into your blood stream. It is possible to eat a nutrient-rich diet of real foods *and still* be nutrient deficient because of poor digestive health.[4]

Without a healthy balance of bacteria and yeast in your gut, you risk experiencing a host of nervous disorders including mood disorders, ADD, & autism, as well as autoimmune disorders like type 1 diabetes, irritable-bowel syndrome, and multiple sclerosis.[5]

So how do you know if you're in good digestive health or not?

First, you'll want to ask yourself some rather obvious questions. I say "obvious," but really so many of us live with digestive complaints daily that we hardly think of them as complaints. For example, do you get gas after eating meals? Do you often have the need to burp after eating? Do you get in-

Bristol Stool Chart

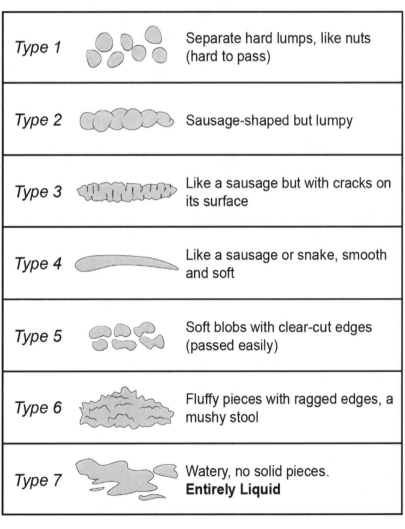

Type 1		Separate hard lumps, like nuts (hard to pass)
Type 2		Sausage-shaped but lumpy
Type 3		Like a sausage but with cracks on its surface
Type 4		Like a sausage or snake, smooth and soft
Type 5		Soft blobs with clear-cut edges (passed easily)
Type 6		Fluffy pieces with ragged edges, a mushy stool
Type 7		Watery, no solid pieces. **Entirely Liquid**

digestion or heartburn after eating meals? Do you have any noticeable food intolerances? Can you eat dairy or grains without much complaint? Do you have a bowel movement at least once per day?

You can also tell quite a bit from your bowel movements. Again, this should be obvious, but so many of us lean towards constipation or diarrhea on a routine basis that our definitions of those words is actually quite murky.

The Bristol Stool Chart was first developed by researchers at the University of Bristol in 1997, and is used to help people identify the exact quality of their stool.[6]

Stools at the lumpy end of the scale like types 1 and 2 are hard to pass, usually requiring a lot of straining. Stools at the loose or liquid end of the continuum like types 5, 6, and 7 can be too easy to pass—the need to pass them is urgent and accidents can happen. The ideal stools are types 3 and 4, especially type 4, as they are most likely to glide out without any delay, straining, or discomfort.

If you aren't routinely passing type 3 or 4 stools, then something is wrong with your digestion. Your gut is probably responding to toxins, stress, or foods in a harmful way.

After this cursory look at your digestive health, you may want to dig deeper. Because your digestive health and mental health are so closely linked, you may want to ask yourself about various mental and nervous disorders. Have you been diagnosed with any mood disorders? ADD? Autism? Do you suffer from any autoimmune disorders like type 1 diabetes, irritable-bowel syndrome, or multiple sclerosis? If you answer yes to any of these, I'd be willing to bet money that you also suffer from gut *dysbiosis*.

Finally, ask yourself if you've got any of these major risk factors for gut *dysbiosis*:

Were you born via a cesarean section instead of vaginally? Our initial gut population is picked up as we pass out the birth canal, so our mother's bacterial milieu becomes our own.[7]

Did you ever take a course of antibiotics without intentionally replacing the good bacteria those antibiotics killed? Antibiotics kill our inner microbial life indiscriminately, wiping out good bacteria along with the harmful pathogens causing our illness, permanently altering our microbiome.[8 9 10]

Do you eat a diet high in sugar and starches? These foods feed the bad bacteria and yeast in your gut, helping them to out-compete the good bacteria and yeast.[11]

Do you drink or bathe in unfiltered water full of heavy metals, chlorine, or chloramines? These toxins are known anti-microbials or disinfectants that have no problem killing off the good bacteria in your gut.[12 13]

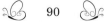

Did you ever routinely take hormonal birth control? Your gut flora is partially responsible for the metabolism of female sex hormones.[14] Artificial hormones can disrupt the balance of your gut flora.[15]

In recent years, a few diets have been prescribed by doctors and researchers to help heal gut disorders. A few of the more prominent healing diets include the Gut And Psychology Syndrome Diet (also known as GAPS), the Body Ecology Diet, and the Specific Carbohydrate Diet (also known as SCD). Many also find improvement without implementing any sort of healing protocol, they just eliminate the problem causing food groups from their diets. Some of the more popular of these diets include the Gluten-Free and/or Casein-Free Diet, the Paleo Diet, and the Primal Diet.

If you're not sure yet whether or not one of these diets is best for you, you should at least make sure you're eating a diet that promotes gut health.

To keep the right balance of bacteria thriving in your digestive tract, do the following:

Avoid sugar and starches

Bad bacteria thrive on sugar. It is their food of choice. You shouldn't eat *any* refined sugars like table sugar or high-fructose corn syrup, and you should greatly reduce the amount of starches you eat (think: corn, potatoes, grains, legumes). If you are willing to properly prepare grains and legumes via soaking, sprouting, or fermenting, they should be fine unless you have some underlying hormonal or digestive issue.

Eat the right balance of omega-6 to omega-3 fats

Too many omega-6 fatty acids can lead to inflammation and exacerbate digestive problems. A *huge* step in this direction can be made if you eliminate seed-based yellow cooking oils (corn oil, soybean oil, vegetable oil, canola oil, etc.) from your diet and begin cooking with more the more traditional fats outlined in the last chapter. Try to eat foods naturally rich in omega-3 fats like wild-caught seafood at least twice per week. You'll also want to eat meats and dairy from wild or pasture-fed animals.

Avoid trans fats

It almost seems silly saying it because it's so obvious. Trans fats hide in all sorts of foods, even those labeled "trans-fat free" thanks to our shoddy labeling laws, which allow foods with less than 0.5g of trans fat per serving to still claim 0g of trans fats per serving. To eliminate these from your diet, you'll need to avoid any foods containing partially-hydrogenated oils and

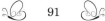

any foods fried in yellow seed-based vegetable oils (i.e. French fries at your local fast food chain), etc.

Eat more soups & stocks

As you learned in the last chapter, homemade stocks from animal bones and cartilage are excellent at promoting digestive health and healing the intestinal lining.

Supplement with probiotics and fermented cod liver oil

Although I'm not a huge fan of supplements, these are the two biggest exceptions to my rule. These two supplements combine to form a veritable powerhouse that promotes intestinal healing. Probiotics help repopulate the gut with good bacteria while the omega-3s and vitamins A & D in the fermented cod liver oil help reduce inflammation and supply the gut with what it needs to heal.

Eat more fermented and living foods

This is, without a doubt, the single greatest thing you can do for your gut health. And, for those of us eating a modern diet, it can also be one of the most confusing.

Just take Melanie for an example. One day, she and I met up for a lunch date at a favorite local restaurant. She sat across the table from me enviously eying my salad. "I'd really love some vegetables right now," she said. We started talking about her diet—the typical diet of the typical American.

I told her that 60-80% of the diet of traditional people groups isn't cooked. "Oh," she interrupted, "I bet I don't cook 60% of the food I eat."

She missed my point. She was talking about sandwiches and cold breakfast cereals, snack bars and mozzarella cheese sticks. Let's not beat around the bush, people. The Standard American Diet *is cooked*. Aside from the occasional salad or piece of fruit, we just don't eat raw foods. In fact, we fear them.

Before the era of refrigeration, eating fermented and living food was part and parcel of a typical diet. Now, I bet you'd be hard-pressed to name something fermented that isn't alcohol. (And even that, we usually pasteurize.)

If I asked you to name a fermented food, what would you pick? Sauerkraut? Kimchi? Chutney? Did you even think of cheese, sour cream, yogurt, sourdough bread or buttermilk pancakes?

Traditional food cultures also relied heavily on raw animal foods.[16] Don't get all squeamish on me. Think. Maybe you've tried some of these traditional dishes before. Have you ever eaten corned beef? That's just raw brisket rolled in salt and spices until it cures. Pastrami? That's just corned beef that's been smoked, usually at a temperature low enough that the meat is still considered raw. (A food is only considered cooked if it's internal temperature is raised above 118°F.) Ceviche? That's raw seafood like shrimp or fish that's been soaked in lemon or limejuice with added tomatoes, peppers, and cilantro. Because these foods are all "cooked" with salt or something acidic rather than heat, they're chock full of beneficial bacteria and enzymes.

Other traditional raw animal foods are harder for some of us to stomach, perhaps because we *know* they're raw. Unlike the foods above, their flavor and texture are distinctly different from cooked animal foods. Steak tartare, sushi, and even raw (unpasteurized) milk come to mind.

Every culture has a long tradition of fermented and raw foods—foods that provide for healthy intestinal flora and decrease the load on your pancreas and liver.

Sadly, because of today's industrial food model, these traditional foods have morphed into something unrecognizable. Often, corned beef is no longer raw and preserved with salt and spices. Cheeses that used to be made from raw milk are almost always made from devitalized pasteurized milk. Bread makers rarely use real fermented sourdough starters in their so-called sourdough loafs, instead adding enough sourdough culture to give a sour flavor while still using baker's yeast to help the bread rise. And homemakers hardly ever preserve cabbage or cucumbers by fermenting them in a salty brine until they turn into sauerkraut or pickles.

The modern equivalents of age-old fermented foods are nutritionally empty when compared to their historical counterparts. All the beneficial bacteria are dead—eradicated by pasteurization or cooking. If you're body isn't getting this steady supply of concentrated, good bacteria, you're far more likely to develop gut *dysbiosis*.[17]

Fermented foods pre-date refrigerators, hot water bath canning, and modern preservatives. They are one of the ways traditional food cultures "put up" their summer harvest for the winter. Every continent has examples of these naturally fermented foods. There are vegetable ferments like sauerkraut and dill pickles in Europe, kimchi in Asia, kvass in Russia, cortido in the Americas. There are dairy ferments like yogurt, kefir, sour cream, and cheeses. We even have a tradition of preserving our meat through lactic acid fermentation in old-fashioned brine curing of sausages, hams, and even bacon.

The basic premise behind these traditional fermented foods is this: Lacto-bacillus bacteria cultures take over the food, producing lactic acid. This not only increases the nutritional value of the food (often increasing vita-

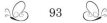

min content like B12 and C by 300-600%!), but it also preserves the food for months or even years while producing a pleasantly sour taste.

In modern, industrialized food production we fear the inconsistency of such traditional natural ferments, so we mimic that sour taste with vinegar while killing off all bacteria using hot water bath or high-pressure canning methods. While this gives us food that tastes almost like the traditional good stuff (or at least it tastes sour), it also gives us dead food devoid of the extra nutrients and healthy beneficial probiotic cultures found in a living, naturally fermented food.

So, if you want to ensure that your nutrient-rich diet isn't going to waste, take care of your gut! Begin introducing more of these living foods into your diet. Don't shy away from traditional raw animal foods or foods that have been cultured with lactic-acid producing bacteria. These foods will repopulate your gut with the good bacteria and enzymes your body needs to properly digest the foods you're eating.

Chapter 6
Eating For Fertility and Pregnancy

As we learned in the second chapter, it was common for traditional fertility diets to begin at least six full months prior to conception. This practice not only increases fertility, but also helps ease mothers through first-trimester maladies like morning sickness, cravings, and food aversions.

That's because these problems have their root cause in mild nutrient-deficiencies.

Unfortunately, if you are already suffering from these common pregnancy afflictions, there is little that you can do to stop them. That's because it takes time to rebuild your body's nutrient stores—more time than the few weeks you have remaining in your first trimester (at which point most of these maladies seem to "magically" go away and resolve themselves). You may, however, be able to ease your symptoms through dietary changes.

If, however, you aren't pregnant yet, consider this your guide to giving yourself the best possible chance for avoiding these uncomfortable and discouraging complaints.

In this chapter, you'll learn about what traditional fertility diets have in common. You'll also learn about what nutritional deficiencies contribute to or cause morning sickness, cravings, food aversions, varicose veins, swelling, pre-eclampsia, and more.

The good news is that the same diet that will increase your fertility will also ease your pregnancy, improve your baby's health, and promote healthy lactation. So, rather than learning a different diet for each phase of the fertility cycle, you'll simply have to familiarize yourself with a few core principles.

In traditional food cultures, Dr. Price noted that women (& men!) ate a diet ten times higher in fat-soluble vitamins than the standard Westerner.[1] They also turned to "sacred foods" when preparing themselves for conception and birth. These sacred foods were even more rich in many vital nutrients, including vitamins A, D, E, and K, as well as DHA, arachadonic acid, choline, biotin, and the entire complex of B vitamins, most notably folate.

The Maasai tribe in Africa, for example, only allowed men and women to marry after spending several months consuming milk from the wet season when the grass was especially lush and the milk much more nutrient-dense. Maasai milk is five times richer in choline than modern supermarket milk

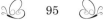

and much higher in fat-soluble vitamins, conjugated linoleic acid (CLA) and omega-3 fatty acids.[2]

In Chapter 2, I argued that the key to giving your children a higher "genetic momentum" is eating a diet rich in methyl-donating nutrients during pregnancy and the first two years of life since these are the nutrients that make it possible to turn on and off genetic expression. As it turns out, the biggest methyl-donating foods are high in Vitamins B12 and B6 and folate. The *best* sources of B12 are shellfish like oysters & claims, followed by liver, fish roe, and other seafood like crab & lobsters, then cheese & eggs. For B6, you can look to liver, tuna, salmon, cod, and brown rice. For folate, we can concentrate on liver, dark leafy greens, and sunflower seeds. Is it any surprise that these foods formed the foundation for traditional fertility diets?

I have to confess, looking at these traditional diets can be a little bit intimidating. There is no way my husband is going to go fishing and bring me back fish heads stuffed with chopped fish liver! And oysters? How many of us regularly eat those? And as much as I admire the regal beauty of the Maasai, I'm not going to subsist on raw milk and animal blood alone.

That's why I was thankful to discover the dietary guidelines established by the Weston A. Price Foundation. Based on Dr. Price's observations about the typical nutrient content of these preconception diets, the Weston A. Price Foundation has created a set of dietary goals for women wishing to conceive. Because it was already in line with so many of the ways I was eating, it wasn't too hard for me to implement. These recommendations have been particularly crafted to fit the taste and inclinations of most Westerners while still being rich in the "sacred foods" essential for fertility, pregnancy, and a growing baby.

Eat According to the Weston A. Price Fertility and Pregnancy Diet

DAILY:

- Supplement with enough fermented cod liver oil to supply 20,000 IU of vitamin A

- Drink 1 quart of whole milk daily, preferably raw and from pasture-fed cows

- 2 or more eggs daily, preferably from pastured chickens

- Additional egg yolks daily, added to smoothies, salad dressings, scrambled eggs, etc.

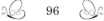

- 2 tbsp. of coconut oil daily, used in cooking or in smoothies
- 4 tbsp. of butter daily, preferably from pasture-fed cows
- Fresh beef or lamb daily, always consumed with the fat
- A cup or more of bone broth, either to drink or used in soups, stews, or sauces
- Lacto-fermented vegetables, condiments, and beverages

WEEKLY:

- 3-5 ounces of liver, once or twice a week
- Fresh seafood, 2-4 times per week, particularly wild salmon, fish eggs, mollusks, and shellfish

Are any of the recommended foods in this diet out of bounds for you because of dietary restrictions or taste preferences? If it's about taste, I'd encourage you to experiment. I've got a recipe section at the back of this book highlighting different ways to prepare and enjoy these sacred foods. Hopefully, something there will inspire you.

If you have dietary restrictions that may prevent you from consuming some of these foods, just remember this rule of thumb. In Dr. Price's survey, people did well so long as they consumed two of these three foods on a regular basis: raw or fermented dairy from pasture-raised animals, fish organs and nutrient-dense seafood, or animal organs from pasture-raised animals. If any of the foods from the diet suggested here is out of the scope of possibility for you, just try to focus on getting 2 out of these 3 foods into your diet daily. Do be aware, however, that if you avoid dairy you need to get your calcium from added bone broth. That's because calcium is a critical nutrient for pregnancy, and without enough of it you're likely to suffer cramps in your hands or feet.

You Want Me to Eat What?

LIVER

Now, before you run away screaming, upset that you've invested this much time and energy reading a book that tells you to eat liver(!) of all things, let me give you a few tips for working liver into your diet that you may not have thought of trying.

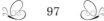

Liver is one of the most nutrient-dense organmeats, yet it's also one of the hardest for most people to stomach. In your diet for preconception, pregnancy, and breastfeeding, you'll want to eat one three to five ounce serving of liver per week (if not more!).

If you have problems with the flavor of liver, here are some suggestions:

- Take your raw liver from grass-fed cows, cut it into pill-sized portions, then freeze them for at least fourteen days (which helps kill any pathogens that may be lurking in the meat). Now you can take your homemade "pills". Each day, take these with a glass of water like you would pills, portioning them out so that you're getting a serving of liver over a period of a week. You get all the benefit of the liver, but without having to "eat" it!

- Hide liver in the midst of ground beef. This works especially well when the ground meat is part of a rich, well-seasoned sauce (like a pasta sauce, soup, or chili). Simply replace 20-25% of the ground meat with ground liver. You honestly can't taste it! To get ground liver: when you buy liver from the butcher, simply ask the man at the counter to grind it. Alternatively, you can use a meat grinder at home. If you don't have a meat grinder, you can grate frozen (slightly thawed) liver using a cheese grater or a food processor.

- Try organ meat sausages! Traditional bologna, Homemade Braunschweiger (p. 195), and liverwurst all contain liver.

- Make paté. It's best to start with Chicken Liver Paté (p. 193), as that can be made quite rich and buttery. The herbal, buttery goodness does an excellent job hiding any liver taste.

FISH ROE

Fish eggs, also known as caviar or roe, can be expensive. It's why most of us Westerners think of it as a luxury food, best served to those with "elevated" or "refined" tastes. That said, some roe, like whitefish roe, is comparatively cheap. I buy it at my local grocery store and pay about $2.50 per ounce. That may sound like a lot, but consider that one ounce contains eight grams of protein and 873 milligrams of omega-3 fats. Plus one mere ounce also contains 54% of the RDA for vitamin B12! In other words, this food is really nutrient-dense, so you don't need to eat a lot of it. A two ounce jar of roe will usually last me for a week of snacking.

If you haven't had roe before, you'll discover that it's usually jarred in lemon juice and salt to act as a preservative. This makes it very flavorful, and a great replacement for salt in some common snacks or dips.

Here are a few of my favorite ways to eat roe:

- Lightly sprinkled over a hard-boiled egg that's been cut in half, lengthwise.
- Stirred into egg salad, tuna salad, or chicken salad.
- Inside meat-and-cheese roll-ups. We'll take a thin slice of meat (usually uncured salami or ham), top it with a slice of cheese or a homemade pimento cheese spread, and then add a dash of roe. Roll it up for an easy, protein-rich snack!
- With smoked salmon and cream cheese.
- Sprinkled over sushi rolls.
- Slightly larger roe varieties (like salmon or trout) are great scrambled into eggs.
- Blended into sour cream or cream cheese herb dips.

SEAFOOD

The most nutrient-dense seafood are mollusks—oysters, clams, mussels, scallops, octopus, and squid. Mollusks are followed by shellfish—lobsters, crayfish, shrimp, or crabs. Fish itself is not particularly nutrient-dense, but a general rule is that the oilier a fish is, the more healthy omega-3 fats you'll be getting. So sardines and anchovies rule the day, although most of us would probably prefer salmon.

You'll want to include seafood in your diet at least three times per week. While that may sound intimidating if you don't eat much seafood, it can actually be done quite casually. I'll typically let at least one lunch be a quick seafood meal (like crab salad or smoked salmon), so that leaves two dinners to plan. A soup like clam chowder is a nice way to incorporate more broth into your diet. Salad shrimp can be tossed into a stir-fry. Scallops can be pan-seared with bacon and lime for a lovely main dish. Salmon can be turned into patties, fish tacos, or served as fillets.

For even more ideas on how to incorporate these nutrient-dense fertility foods into your diet, check out the Recipe Section of this book.

Eat to Prevent Morning Sickness

Nothing is more of a bane to a newly pregnant mother's existence than morning sickness. Eat too much or too little, and suddenly you're hunched over a toilet puking your brains out. Over the years, researchers have developed a number of promising theories about what causes morning sickness. The bottom line is this: The science disagrees.

But, I don't think it has to. After doing a little bit of research of my own, I developed a theory that unifies the best parts of the more reasonable theories out there. I like it. It's simple. It fits with what we know about mild nutritional deficiencies and how various nutrients in our body interact. Plus, it explained a few mysteries—like why morning sickness is more prevalent in the winter. I've passed this theory on to others, along with my advice for how to prevent morning sickness in a nutrition course that I teach online to couples trying to conceive. So far it's worked!

So, here are the most common theories circulating about what causes morning sickness:

Morning sickness protects baby from toxins

According to this theory, morning sickness is good for you. It was evolution's way of making sure that toxins stayed far away from the baby. So, if you get morning sickness, you should count yourself lucky. It means your body's functioning the way it should and is a sign of a healthy pregnancy. It's unfortunate that it's uncomfortable, but you should embrace it as the safety net that it is.

This is the only theory I find intellectually unsettling—mostly because it's just not true to experience. I've known plenty of mothers who eat the most amazing, nutrient-rich, toxin-free diets. They filter the chlorine out of their water. They don't use nasty soaps or chemical detergents. They've bought into the organic lifestyle more strictly than even I have. And, the so-called toxic foods that are making them nauseous? Grass-fed beef, eggs from pastured hens, wild-caught Alaskan salmon. These foods are far from toxic!

I've also known plenty of mothers, like myself, who never experienced any morning sickness at all, yet had a perfectly healthy pregnancy. Some of these moms even ate total junk. I'm talking the kind of food that's brimming with chemical ingredients and other toxins. Why have they never had morning sickness, if the whole purpose is to keep these toxins away from the developing baby?

Morning sickness is the result of your body adjusting to a flood of extra hormones

It is certainly true that your body produces a lot more hormones when pregnant. You've got human chorionic gonadotropin (hCG), which doubles every two days for the first 10 weeks or so of your pregnancy. Progesterone positively skyrockets. Since it's been known to cause drowsiness on par with sleeping tablets, it's no wonder moms are so interminably fatigued during their first trimester. Plus you've got extra estrogen, oxytocin, and relaxin swimming through your veins, among others.

However, I think this theory is incomplete. It doesn't explain, for example, why some women respond poorly to these surging hormones with nausea and morning sickness while others appear to have no symptoms at all.

Morning sickness is caused by low blood sugar

Given that regulating blood sugar by eating frequent meals (and even sometimes in the middle of the night) really helps some women cope with morning sickness, I'm willing to believe this is true. But, I also believe that the low blood sugar is a symptom of what really causes morning sickness, not necessarily a cause in and of itself.

Morning sickness is caused by a deficiency in vitamins B12 and B6

Again, given that many mothers find relief from morning sickness by intentionally eating foods rich in B vitamins or taking B vitamin supplements, I'm willing to believe this is true. But, as above, I think this is a side effect of what really causes morning sickness.

So, what really causes morning sickness? What's my unifying theory? What could possibly be improved by eating more B vitamins *and* keeping your blood sugar even that *also* explains why some women respond so poorly to surging hormones?

Magnesium

Even those of us eating a nutrient dense diet can have a hard time getting enough magnesium in our daily fare. Not too terribly long ago, you could get enough magnesium simply by eating a varied diet and drinking your mineral rich well or spring water.

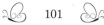

These days, we drink and bathe in water provided by our local cities. These cities treat the water we drink to remove all kinds of undesirables—everything from pharmaceuticals to pesticides. Unfortunately, the unintended side effect of our municipal water treatments is that many of the desirable trace minerals like magnesium, sulfur, and selenium are also removed.

To make matters worse, many opt to "soften" their water by removing "hard" minerals like magnesium.

It's not impossible to get enough magnesium in your diet, but it isn't surprising if you don't.

But I've had my blood levels tested, and I don't have a magnesium deficiency

Perhaps you do. Perhaps you don't. In her book, *The Magnesium Miracle*, Dr. Carolyn Dean answers that objection with this interesting nugget:

> "There has been no lab test that will give an accurate reading of the magnesium status in the tissues. Only one percent of magnesium of the body is distributed in the blood, making a simple sample of magnesium in the blood highly inaccurate. That's why most doctors who rely on blood tests for magnesium—and not magnesium deficiency signs and symptoms—will miss an important diagnosis."[3]

What does a lack of magnesium have to do with morning sickness? How does a lack of magnesium initiate the perfect storm of low blood sugar levels, explain the need for more B vitamins, and reveal why some women respond poorly to surging pregnancy hormones while others don't?

Well, it turns out that one of the primary ways your body uses magnesium is to support adrenal health and regulate cortisol levels. Too much magnesium in your system won't affect normal levels, but a deficiency of magnesium will allow high levels of cortisol to linger. So what's the big deal about that?

Cortisol is your stress hormone. It prompts your body into dumping more sugar into your bloodstream to help you cope with stress. If your cortisol levels stay unnaturally elevated because of a lack of magnesium, your blood sugar will rise . . . and rise . . . and rise. This spike in blood sugar will cause a spiked insulin response, which will then radically decrease your blood sugar levels, often to the other extreme. This, in turn, stresses you out, makes you anxious and nauseous, and can lead to vomiting. Of course this stress prompts your body to once again build up cortisol levels, and without enough magnesium to help you regulate those cortisol levels, you'll enter

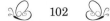

into a vicious, self-perpetuating cycle unless you make a conscious effort to regulate your blood sugar levels through diet.[4]

Even if you don't have a magnesium deficiency before getting pregnant, you can still get one soon thereafter because of the excess flood of pregnancy hormones in your system. That's because those hormones compete for magnesium with the rest of your body! Progesterone, for example, requires both vitamin B6 and magnesium for its synthesis. And as estrogen levels rise, it actually prevents the absorption of magnesium.[5]

With your newly pregnant body making all these increased demands for magnesium, it makes sense that women who supplement with B vitamins can experience some relief. After all, B vitamins are necessary for magnesium absorption! When you increase your B vitamin intake, you automatically increase your absorption of magnesium.[6]

Putting these puzzle pieces together decades before I ever did, the obstetrician George M. Wolverton started treating patients who complained of morning sickness with injections of high doses of B12, B6, and magnesium. In the course of 1,800 pregnancies, he never once saw a woman have to be hospitalized with *hyperemesis gravidarum* (an extreme form of morning sickness). This, when the nationwide average for pregnant mothers diagnosed with HG is roughly 2%.[7] And, he reported that most women experienced relief from morning sickness quickly once supplementation began.[8]

So, how can you prevent morning sickness?

You'll need build up your magnesium stores *before* you get pregnant. That's because, like vitamin D, magnesium takes a while to accumulate, particularly if you're running on empty. If depleted magnesium stores are your norm, it can take as many as four to six weeks before you'll see any noticeable sign of improvement. Give yourself at least three to six months to elevate your levels fully.

If you're already pregnant, you can ameliorate your symptoms with added magnesium, but you may not be able to eliminate your morning sickness altogether.

Foods rich in magnesium include bone broth, leafy green vegetables, properly soaked seeds and nuts, unrefined sea salt and soaked or sprouted whole-grains.

But to really see your magnesium absorption soar, you'll want to also boost those vitamins that are essential for absorption, like B6 and B12. That means eating plenty of shellfish, liver, fish roe, salmon, cod, crab, cheese, and eggs. Vitamin D and calcium are also necessary for magnesium absorption.[9] This is why many moms experience their worst morning sickness during

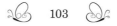

the darker months of late winter. Pregnant mothers who spent their spring, summer and early fall outdoors in the sun got plenty of vitamin D to help shore up their magnesium levels.

If you suffer from any signs of magnesium deficiency like constipation, irritability, anxiety, weight gain, low thyroid function, restless leg syndrome, foggy thinking, or insomnia, you may want to consider attacking the deficiency head on with supplementation in addition to an improved diet. Magnesium is one of those minerals that's best absorbed through the skin rather than orally.[10] Because of this, I personally choose to apply magnesium oil to my skin rather than take some pills.

What if you already have morning sickness?

• *Start supplementing immediately with magnesium oil*

Rub it onto your skin liberally and often. I recommend the Ancient Minerals brand of magnesium oil. To figure out your dose, simply pay attention to your poop! Magnesium will help loosen your stools. If you get diarrhea, you are using too much magnesium. If, however, you're simply getting a nice, soft stool and avoiding constipation, then you're probably using enough.

• *Get more sun!*

By this, I mean real sunlight, direct, in the middle of the day, with limbs and belly exposed. Sitting behind glass windows sadly does not offer the same benefits, since most glass blocks the UVB rays necessary to create vitamin D in your skin but let the vitamin D-leaching UVA rays through.

• *Take more fermented cod liver oil*

Magnesium absorption is dependent on the presence of vitamin D, so if you can't get out in the sun enough, be sure to take extra fermented cod liver oil. Fermented cod liver oil is a food that's rich in vitamins A, D, K, and omega-3 fatty acids. If fermented cod liver oil also makes you want to gag, then...

• *Supplement with Standard Process vitamins*

Weston A. Price Foundation board member and practicing physician Dr. Tom Cowan recommends supplementing during pregnancy with a multi-vitamin that can help fill critical nutrient gaps. The multi-vitamin he recom-

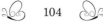

mends is Catalyn by Standard Process. It is rich in magnesium and vitamins D, A, and B6. He also recommends Cataplex B12 by Standard Process. Along with Vitamin D, B6 and B12 are also essential for proper absorption of magnesium. Standard Process makes whole food based supplements and does not use synthetically created vitamins or minerals at all.

• *Eat before you get out of bed*

Since low blood sugar levels will make your nausea worse, it is best to try to keep your blood sugar level as even as possible. Keep hard cheese, apples, bananas, and nuts by your bed. Snack on them when you get up in the middle of the night to pee, and then again when you first wake up.

• *Eat more frequently*

Again, since low blood sugar levels will make your nausea worse, try eating smaller, more frequent meals throughout the day. Never go more than 2 or 3 hours without eating.

• *Try to eat more protein and saturated fat*

Notice the word "try." If you already have morning sickness, chances are you also already have the food aversions and cravings that go with it.

That also means that the idea of eating eggs from pastured hens, a juicy steak, or a pot roast may be making you nauseated. Why is that? It's obvious your body needs these foods, as they will help keep your blood sugar levels even while providing your body with what it needs to build hormones, blood volume, and more. But you still get a little sick just reading about them, let alone actually smelling them on your dinner plate.

If you find that your first-trimester body is rejecting fatty and protein-rich foods and craving carbohydrates, here's why. It has to do with cholesterol. Hormones are made from cholesterol, and your pregnant body is making *a lot* of extra hormones right now. But your liver also uses cholesterol to create the bile it needs to help digest fats. Your pregnant body is wisely putting a priority on creating those pregnancy hormones, which means it doesn't have enough cholesterol left to digest fatty foods. Thankfully, your body has a workaround. It can create cholesterol from carbohydrates! While this is fine as a stopgap measure, it's far from ideal. That's because a diet of fried potatoes and waffles simply isn't rich in the protein, B vitamins, and fat-soluble vitamins A, D, E, and K that you need.

So, even if you find you have aversions to these fatty foods, you should still try to get more protein and fats into your diet. You may find relief by supplementing with bitters and/or ox bile to help your liver digest these necessary nutrients. Standard Process also makes a supplement with this exact combination of bitters and bile salts to aid in fat digestion called Cholacol. You can also support your liver by drinking Milk Thistle Tea.

- *If you're having trouble keeping anything at all down, sip on raw milk or bone broth throughout the day*

Raw milk and bone broth are often the only foods a mother suffering from morning sickness can tolerate. Plus, they also happen to be rich in calcium—a mineral that works synergistically with magnesium within the body. Since calcium competes with magnesium for absorption within the body, supplementing with high levels of magnesium to correct that deficiency may inadvertently create a calcium deficiency. Thus, it is wonderfully helpful to increase consumption of both together, particularly if your intake of calcium would already have been low.

Remember, if you are already suffering from morning sickness, you are not likely to alleviate your symptoms completely. But you can make them far more manageable by immediately giving your body what it needs most right now—magnesium, vitamins D, B6, and B12, and steady blood sugar levels.

Eat to Prevent Swelling and Varicose Veins

If morning sickness, food aversions, and food cravings mark the first trimester of pregnancy, swelling ankles and varicose veins mark the last. Those middle few months? Most moms say they're like the eye of a hurricane, the calm before the storm. They feel energetic and downright radiant.

Thankfully, you can avoid the swelling and varicose veins of your last trimester easily if you implement a few pieces of dietary advice from Dr. Thomas Brewer.

Dr. Brewer is the OBGYN who discovered the cause of pre-eclampsia, a condition of late pregnancy where mothers experience high blood pressure and excess protein in the urine. He blamed abnormal blood volume levels caused by poor nutrition, and prescribed a diet very sympathetic to the traditional fertility and pregnancy diets (lots of eggs, milk, liver, and seafood). His goal was to make sure that mothers were getting adequate amounts of protein (between 80 grams and 120 grams per day), enough calories (to make sure they actually used all that protein, as a low-calorie diet in combination with a high-protein diet causes the body to go into ketosis and pee all that wonderful protein away), and enough salt (so that the mother's liver and kidneys could function optimally).[11]

Like the frame of a house, proteins hold your body together. Your body uses proteins to build, well to build *you.*

Yes, the tissues of your muscle are made of protein, but structural proteins also hold together just about every other part of your body, too. Although bone is predominantly calcium, that calcium is held together in a composite made up of protein. Your nerves are mostly made of fats, but protein is the framework that holds nerves together. Blood vessels, organs, and skin all have structural proteins.

For example, as you age, collagen (a supporting protein in your skin) breaks down. Lacking the structural support, your skin wrinkles and sags. Indeed just about everything about you is made of protein. Your hair, your nails, and your hormones are also protein. Did you know your body contains some ten thousand to fifty thousand kinds of protein?

These proteins are constantly being broken down into amino acids, recycled and built anew, even burned to provide energy. You need to eat protein every day just to sustain life because your body cannot store protein the way it stores fat.

During a healthy pregnancy, you need *even more* protein to build your baby. Your baby needs muscles, bones, nerves, blood vessels, organs, and skin just like you. You also need the extra protein to build your uterus. When the uterus is not pregnant, it weighs only two ounces. Did you know that at the end of a healthy pregnancy, the uterus alone weighs two pounds? This means that you need to grow about one pound and fourteen ounces of new uterine muscle cells with every pregnancy. I'm not even mentioning your placenta, which is usually equal in size, or the four pounds of extra blood that will be circulating through your veins!

If you don't give your body enough protein to build a baby, build up your uterus, and built an entirely new organ from scratch while also maintaining all your current organs, bones, and blood vessels, swelling and varicose veins are the result. Your body will prioritize the baby, which means your own cellular structure is weakened. Whenever the capillary lining is *weak,* the leakage of *protein* across the *capillary walls* into the interstitial space results in swelling. And, when the capillaries eventually break from the extra pressure, they leave small blood marks under the skin. The veins themselves can become swollen, painful and distorted. Hence, varicose veins.

Some people feel that Dr. Brewer's pregnancy diet is too high in protein, that it's dangerous. When asked what the upper limit for protein consumption in pregnancy should be, birth educator and Brewer Pregnancy Diet advocate Joy Jones, R.N. said:

"Nobody knows, but it certainly isn't the 45 to 60 grams a day some writers propose. In very carefully controlled research at the University of California at Berkeley, for instance, pregnant women were fed diets that contained varying levels of protein—up to 120 grams a day—and it was found that their bodies were still using the protein even at the highest levels of intake.

The theory behind the thinking of those who are leery of protein is that when you eat large amounts of protein, you create a higher level of metabolic by-products that the liver and kidneys must clear from the body. The fear is that the by-products will overpower the body's ability to handle them. This line of reasoning misses an important point: When you have a completely adequate diet, the liver and kidneys get their share of essential nutrients and so step up their clearance rate with no difficulty whatever. In short, you can't overdose on the levels of protein this diet provides—and probably not at levels significantly higher, either."[12]

So, how can you get enough protein?

When people plan on eating more protein, their first thought is: more steak! More roast! More meat! But I've found it's easy to get burned out on red meat. So here's what I've done in the past to keep my pregnancy protein levels topping 80-120 grams per day.

- *Eat at least two eggs per day*

Eggs are the perfect breakfast food. They can be poached and served with hollandaise sauce (a way to get extra yolks, YAY!), fried in coconut oil, scrambled with leftover meats and vegetables, or blended into yogurt or kefir smoothies. When you're tired of eggs for breakfast, try eggs for lunch or dinner instead. I love egg salad made with bacon grease, mayonnaise, salt, & pepper. I also really love a quiche cooked up with Swiss cheese and fried rice made with eggs & shrimp. Try to stick to eggs from pasture-raised hens.

Consider that there are six grams of protein per egg, for a total of twelve grams per day. Each additional egg yolk also contains three additional grams of protein.

• Drink at least one quart (four cups) of whole milk per day

Of course, this milk is preferably raw and from pasture-fed cows. Each cup contains eight grams of protein, for a total of thirty-two grams of protein per day.

• Chicken, salmon, tuna, and crab are your friends

These all make great salads when blended with mayonnaise or sour cream—especially helpful when you don't have the time, inclination, or energy to cook. I tend to eat four-and-a-half to six ounces of these meats stirred into a salad dressing of mayo. Toss in dried cranberries or apples for a lift, and add a spoonful or two of chopped nuts or seeds to get even more protein.

Six ounces of chicken meat has fifty grams of protein! Six ounces of salmon has 102 grams of protein! Six ounces of tuna has forty-two grams. And six ounces of crabmeat has thirty grams.

• Snack on hard cheeses and nuts

A couple of slices of hard cheese is usually around one ounce (imagine a one-inch cube) and makes a good snack along with a small handful of roasted nuts. Try to stick to grass-fed cheeses.

One ounce of hard cheese has seven or eight grams of protein, as does a small handful of nuts or seeds.

• Don't forget beans, nut butters, yogurt, sprouted grain bread, and cottage cheese!

These are often overlooked sources of protein in a typical diet since they're not meat, eggs, or hard cheese. I was often surprised to remember that a single slice of my sprouted grain bread had seven ounces of protein. So, a tuna melt for lunch could earn me forty-eight grams of protein in one fell swoop.

• Gelatin

Gelatin is protein, so each tablespoon contains anywhere from seven to twelve grams of protein depending on how it was processed and what the source is. I recommend Great Lakes Kosher Gelatin, since it's from grass-fed cows and low-temperature processed to avoid creating free glutamic acids.

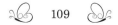

You can stir it into hot beverages (it's tasteless), make desserts like Jell-O or marshmallows, or even add it into a breakfast smoothie. I've even stirred it into my already well-gelled homemade broths just for some extra kick.

Eat to Prevent Stretch Marks

In our culture, we accept stretch marks as a given. We're told by our OB/GYNs that our skin is either elastic, or it isn't. If it's elastic, you get fewer stretch marks. If it's not elastic, you get a belly full of them. And, we're told most women *will get stretch marks*, no matter what they do to try to prevent them.

Well guess what? You can prevent stretch marks.

Wanna know how? By increasing the elasticity of your skin! And that's done through (you guessed it!) nutrition.

We've long known that your skin's elasticity, firmness, and functioning are dependent on certain key nutrients. That's why certain vitamin deficiencies cause skin damage, and why supplementing with the depleted nutrients restores skin health.[13]

Yet despite this, very few studies have been done on diet and skin elasticity. A few have been done on diet and wrinkling, or diet and sunburns. But specifically on elasticity? Not so much. This prompted a team of researchers to conduct a study that was published in the 2010 study published in the *British Journal of Nutrition*. They found that skin elasticity significantly improved with a diet higher in saturated and monounsaturated fat, fish oil supplementation, and increased antioxidants.[14] These results are similar to the results of a 2008 study that measured a 10% increase in skin elasticity when women took an oral fish oil supplement,[15] and a 2007 study that showed improved elasticity with an increase in antioxidant consumption.[16]

Fish oil is naturally high in omega-3 fatty acids, so it's safe to say that the extra supplementation may have helped push the dietary intake ratios of omega-6 to omega-3 fats into optimal range. This, of course, would have an anti-inflammatory effect, which in turn reduces free radicals in the skin and helps keep it elastic and firm. The researchers speculated that the higher fat diets contributed to elasticity because maintenance of collagen and elastic fibers requires fat. It also improves the lipid profile of the skin, making it smoother and less dry. And finally, the increased antioxidant intake in vitamins like E, C, and even A would also counter the effect of free radicals, protecting the skin and keeping it elastic.

Perhaps the more obvious reason why vitamin C has a noticeably protective effect on the skin is that you need it for collagen formation. Collagen and skin elasticity go together like peas and carrots. Likewise, gelatin also aides collagen formation. At least one study was done to measure the effects of supplementing with gelatin on skin elasticity, and found measurable improvement.[17] Of course, the best-known food source of gelatin is homemade bone broth, especially those broths made from oxtail or chicken feet. (Yet one more reason to stick like glue to the one cup per day recommendation made by the Weston A. Price foundation!)

What does a diet higher in saturated fat, lower in omega-6 fats, higher in omega-3 fats, higher in gelatin, and rich in the antioxidants vitamins A, C, and E look like?

(You should know the answer by now.)

Why, it's the traditional fertility and pregnancy diet embraced by cultures around the world!

Eat for a Pleasant Birth

The typical hospital birth environment has a strange and unnatural rule: no eating or drinking allowed during labor. Some let you suck on ice cubes or sip water or Gatorade. Most hook you up to an IV early on to keep you from dehydrating. This is because they're prepping you for an emergency surgery (a C-section), and patients are always encouraged to have empty stomachs, purged bowels, and empty bladders before going into surgery. It is not because a lack of food or drink during labor is somehow normal or healthy.

If you eat, it is possible that in the stress of labor you may throw up. If you haven't had a recent bowel movement, it's possible you'll poop while pushing the baby out. The risk of doing either can be greatly minimized simply by using the restroom semi-frequently during labor. So, don't sweat it! Eat your food; drink your drinks. Give your body the fuel it needs to give birth!

First Stage of Labor

The first stage of labor starts when you begin having regular contractions that are growing in intensity and frequency. It ends just before the baby starts moving down the birth canal.

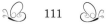

Early Labor

This is when your body is using contractions to open your cervix. It is usually slow and steady. Unless the baby has an awkward presentation, the contractions will feel like surges of pressure building around your abdomen. This is the time to eat!

<u>What should you eat?</u> Whatever you want! Eat heavier foods earlier on so that you have the chance to digest them before labor gets too intense. If your contractions feel intense, stick to lighter foods—fruits, nuts, honey, and cheese slices.

<u>What should you drink?</u> I highly recommend coconut water. It's nature's Gatorade, but without the chemical additives and high-fructose corn syrup. If you don't want coconut water, stick to plain water. Anything else (like milk, tea, soda, or coffee) will adversely affect your digestion or hormones.

Transition

This is the last part of the first stage of labor. In it, your cervix is opening the final stretch necessary to make room for the baby's head to enter the birth canal. This is also the stage of labor where mothers often experience the most scattered thoughts and wild sensations. Even in easy, pain-free labors, mothers may feel like they can't keep enduring, or like they don't know how to cope.

<u>What should you eat or drink?</u> Nothing. If your birth practitioner wants you to keep your fluids up, then sip gently on coconut water or water. Food will be the last thing on your mind anyway. The only reason to eat during this stage is if your labor has stalled here, and you need more energy to keep going. In that case, stick to the lighter foods like bananas, nuts, or cheese slices.

<u>*Second Stage of Labor*</u>

This stage begins when the baby descends into the birth canal and ends when your baby is born. It's often a relieving stage. Each surge of the contractions feels purposeful. Moms have a strong desire to push or breath the baby out (much like the feeling you get before a bowel movement). To minimize tearing, take this phase as slowly as possible to give your skin a chance to stretch around the baby's head. But really, helping your skin get elastic enough to not tear is a matter of nutrition during pregnancy—the same foods that help prevent stretch marks (those rich in vitamins A, B2, B6, C, and E, along with plenty of good saturated fat). It's also affected by hydration, so stay hydrated!

What should you eat or drink? Nothing. If your birth practitioner wants you to keep your fluids up, then sip gently on coconut water or water. Trust me, you won't want to eat anything during these moments anyway.

Third Stage of Labor

This is when you give birth to the placenta. After your baby is born, you can hold it to your chest for a few minutes. Then, as they root around or make suckling noises, you can help them find your nipple and start to nurse. The nipple stimulation will release even more oxytocin—the hormone responsible for bonding, affection, and contractions! The extra contractions are essential for shrinking your uterus, preventing hemorrhaging, and helping your placenta disengage from your uterine wall so that it, too, can be birthed.

What should you eat or drink? Sips of coconut water or water are okay. You'll probably not want to eat at all during this stage and may instead feel nausea.

Fourth Stage of Labor

But wait! There are only three stages! NOT. Just because your baby and placenta are out doesn't mean you're done. You still need to get cleaned up, nurse your baby to sleep, get stitches for any tearing, put on some funky underwear (ugly, but surprisingly comfy), and settle down into bed. And, you'll still be having contractions as your uterus shrinks.

What should you eat or drink? Eat whatever you crave. Stick to something nutrient dense coupled with something full of good carbohydrates. Believe it or not, my favorite afterbirth food is a chocolate smoothie made with raw milk, yogurt, fruit, almond butter, and cocoa. Any foods that are good for recovery from hard workouts will be excellent to eat now! Now you can sip on Mother's Milk Tea by Traditional Medicinals (www.traditionalmedicinals.com/product/mother-s-milk-reg) or drink some raw milk. If you're struggling with nausea or pain, try a few drops of AfterBirth Drops by Native Remedies (www.nativeremedies.com/products/afterbirthdrops-natural-oxytocin-placenta-delivery.html) or some Arnica (which treats shock symptoms).

Chapter 7

Nutritional Myth-Busting

The average pregnant woman is inundated with rules. Don't eat soft cheese. If you eat lunchmeat, reheat it to kill the listeria. Don't change your cat's litter. You absolutely must not drink any alcohol at all. Don't eat fish; you risk exposure to toxic levels of mercury. Avoid raw milk and raw cheeses. Don't drink more than a cup of coffee per day. Don't lie on your back. Don't eat more than 30% of your calories as fat. And, the list goes on.

The rules can be overwhelming. In fact, there are so many of them, many women have started pushing back. I know I did. I wanted to know if there was really anything to these taboos.

Turns out, every culture has a set of taboos. But perhaps even more eye-opening is the idea that these taboos aren't universally shared. For example, in France, doctors encourage pregnant women to not eat raw vegetables! If you're pregnant and eating salad, people will look at you like you've grown a third head. And yet, French culture assumes that pregnant women should drink a glass of red wine per day for health!

So, in this chapter, I've set out to explore some of our culture's most common pregnancy taboos and nutritional myths and separate out the fact from the fiction, using traditional wisdom as my guide.

Are Saturated Fat and Cholesterol Really Bad for You?

Doctors recommend a low-cholesterol, low-saturated fat diet, not only for pregnant women, but for everybody. That's because they believe that diets high in cholesterol and saturated fat put you at risk for heart disease.

Until the advent of the Industrial Revolution, the only fats available for humans to eats were those traditional, healthy fats covered in Chapter 4. Around the turn of the last century, vegetable shortening came on the scene. Solid and shelf-stable like most animal fats, it was billed as a cheaper alternative to lard (by far the world's most popular animal fat at the time). At around the same time, oleomargarine was also invented and sold as imita-

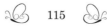

tion butter. Of course, people loved the flavor and texture of lard and butter and considered the vegetable oil alternatives cheap, unhealthy imitations of the real thing. So, only the poor embraced the new fats.

In the 1950s, things started to change. A prominent scientist by the name of Ancel Keys postulated a theory that the amount of saturated fat and cholesterol in the diet was directly correlated to incidence of heart disease. This theory became known as the lipid hypothesis. He published his findings in a book, went on radio and television to promote his theory, and became a nutritional celebrity almost overnight. Keys plotted the average dietary intake of saturated fat for seven different countries on a graph, along with the incidence of heart disease for those countries. The graph showed a strong link between the two. The more saturated fat a society ate, the more heart disease they suffered from.

It wasn't long before others in the scientific community began to point out that the correlation swiftly broke down when you added in data from other countries. In fact, when you consider that Keys had data from more than fifty countries at hand, but only chose to highlight the seven which proved his hypothesis, you may rightfully start to wonder whether he was being as forthright as a scientist should have been.

Yet Keys had a charismatic personality and his own television show, and by 1961, he'd even made the cover of *Time* magazine. So his ideas spread.

People began to turn to yellow-seed-based vegetable oils, margarine, and vegetable shortening to replace the saturated fat in their diets.

In 1968, the U.S. government also got involved when Senator George McGovern convened the Select Committee on Nutrition and Human Needs. Over the following nine years, the committee convened several highly publicized hearings in which vociferous doctors, nutritionists, and scientists debated the ins and outs of the contemporary U.S. diet. In 1977, McGovern published the committee's conclusion: Americans should eat less red meat. The meat industry was in an uproar. You can't say that! You can't just tell Americans to stop buying our meat! So, the committee edited their final conclusion. The one thing that contemporary nutrition science knew about red meat compared to other meats was that it had more saturated fat in it. So, rather than saying Americans should eat less red meat, the report concluded that Americans should eat less saturated fat.

Of course, many scientists, doctors, and nutritionists protested: Wait! There's no link between dietary intake of saturated fat and incidence of heart disease! You can't single out one nutrient and start telling Americans to avoid it.

Too late.

The U.S. Department of Health and Human Services stood by its warning that saturated fat was bad for you. Americans needed to replace these fats with something, so they turned towards modern industrial vegetable oils.

Of course, further research has since shown that the lipid hypothesis is false. Numerous studies followed, with researchers falsely claiming that the conclusions supported the lipid hypothesis. However, a close reading of the actual studies reveals otherwise. For example, quite a few such studies used hydrogenated animal fats as their sample for saturated fats. A fat is hydrogenated when you force extra hydrogen atoms onto the unsaturated fatty acid in order to make it mimic a saturated fatty acid. The primary way to hydrogenate fats creates trans-fats. If trans-fats occur in nature, they are usually only 2% or less of the total fat. When they're created artificially, they can be up to 45% of the total fat. Many of the studies claiming to "prove" the dangers of saturated fats only actually proved the dangers of excess trans fats.

Recently, a number of meta-analysis studies have been released in which scientists combed all the data from all the studies that have ever been done on dietary intake of saturated fat and incidence of heart disease. When scientists do a meta-analysis, it is usually in the hope of finding a statistically significant pool of information to help prove their hypothesis. For example, pretend that 10 studies had been done on diet and incidence of heart disease. Each study only had a hundred participants, so any conclusion about diet and heart disease from that study might be statistically insignificant. But if you pool the results from all ten studies in a meta-analysis, you might be able to demonstrate some statistically significant results.

So, what have the recent meta-analysis studies discovered? That there is no link between dietary intake of saturated fat and incidence of heart disease. Of the recent meta-analysis studies, the two most famous ones were published in prominent journals. The first, titled "A Systematic Review of the Evidence Supporting a Causal Link Between Dietary Factors and Coronary Heart Disease" was published in the 2009 *Archive of Internal Medicine*.[1] The second, titled "Meta-analysis of prospective cohort studies evaluating the association of saturated fat with cardiovascular disease" was published in the January 2010 edition of the *American Journal of Clinical Nutrition*.[2] Dr. Ronald Krauss, the study's principal investigator and director of atherosclerosis research at Children's Hospital Oakland Research Institute, said, "It's time to turn the page on how we perceive saturated fats in relation to risk for heart disease. It's the wrong message that saturated fats are artery-clogging or evil."[3] Krauss says any dietary recommendations to further reduce saturated fat would be of no benefit. Americans, he says, shouldn't be avoiding

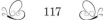

all forms of saturated fats and it's erroneous to focus on saturated fat out of context from the whole diet.

In recent years, we've also come to better understand the role that cholesterol plays within our bodies. Dr. Natasha Campbell-McBride, Ph.D. has introduced it this way:

> "The question is, why do some people have more cholesterol in their blood than others, and why can the same person have different levels of cholesterol at different times of the day? Why is our level of cholesterol different in different seasons of the year? In winter it goes up and in the summer it goes down. Why is it that blood cholesterol goes through the roof in people after any surgery? Why does blood cholesterol go up when we have an infection? Why does it go up after dental treatment? Why does it go up when we are under stress? And why does it become normal when we are relaxed and feel well? The answer to all these questions is this: Cholesterol is a healing agent in the body. When the body has some healing jobs to do, it produces cholesterol and sends it to the site of the damage."[4]

It is true that many people with heart disease show increased levels of cholesterol in their blood, but if we know anything more about cholesterol now than we did a decade or two ago it's this: Cholesterol is the body's "fireman," on the scene to put out fires. It is not, in and of itself, responsible for heart disease.

So, should you be afraid of eating more saturated fat and cholesterol? Absolutely not!

Do You Really Need That Iron Supplement?

The Centers for Disease Control recommends that every pregnant woman take 30 grams of iron daily, and if anemia is suspected, at least twice that. The idea is simple. Mothers need iron to facilitate the growth of the placenta and baby. This much is absolutely true.[5] And a number of studies have drawn connections between mothers who have anemia with low birth weight and premature birth.

What makes iron so pivotal to fetal growth? Two things. First, iron carries oxygen from the lungs to every cell in the body. Second, it makes blood. Your blood volume will increase by at least 50% during pregnancy. This extra blood is used to nourish your placenta and baby. If you don't make

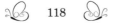

enough blood, or if it doesn't have enough red blood cells to carry adequate amounts of oxygen, your baby can't grow.

Yet does that mean you should supplement with iron? Are all these pregnant women really anemic?

In the U.S., we routinely check a pregnant mother's red blood cell count (hemoglobin) in the belief that this test can effectively detect anemia and iron deficiency. After all, that's the test we use to diagnose anemia in otherwise healthy adults.

Skeptic and fellow mother, Nina Planck, says that for most pregnant women, a diagnosis of anemia is wrong. "The average healthy pregnant woman may have lower hemoglobin, but she is not anemic," Planck explains. "Hemoglobin concentration as low as 9.0 ml/dg in pregnancy is normal, not pathological. It's a side effect of greater blood volume, which is not only normal but essential for a healthy pregnancy."[6]

The idea is that as your blood volume rapidly increases, the presence of hemoglobin in the blood is diluted. This decrease shows up in lab tests that measure the concentration of hemoglobin in the blood, leading doctors to diagnose pregnant mothers with a pregnancy-induced anemia. In fact, the hemoglobin levels only drop temporarily until you can make enough to sustain your greater blood volume.

If lower hemoglobin levels really were an indication of anemia and iron-deficiency, then lower hemoglobin levels would also correlate tightly with birth weight. But they don't. A large British study, involving more than 150,000 pregnancies, found that the highest average birth weight was in the group of women who had low hemoglobin concentrations.[7]

So what if you don't really have anemia? Wouldn't it still be better to err on the side of caution and just take a supplement? That way, your bases are covered.

Unfortunately, most iron supplements aren't made with the same kind of iron that you'd find in food. They're made of inorganic iron salts that cause constipation. As you learned from the last chapter, taking care of your digestion is paramount! You want to be able to absorb the nutrients from all those wonderfully rich, traditional fertility and pregnancy foods you're eating, right? Constipation is a sign of poor digestion, so these non-food iron sources are doing *something* to upset the ecosystem of your gut.

Rather than taking a risky supplement, opt to eat more iron rich foods like red meat, clams, liver, and oysters. Vitamin C helps aide iron's absorption, as does Yellow Dock (a common herbal supplement).

If you must take a supplement, consider using Floradix (www.florahealth.com/product_conditions_usa.cfm?conditions_id=6&prod_id=205),

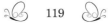

a liquid supplement composed of organic, food sourced iron. Likewise, you may find Ferrofood from Standard Process (www.standardprocess.com/Products/Standard-Process/Ferrofood) helpful. Both of these are food-based supplements that use organic, rather than inorganic, iron.

Will I Really Get Listeria from That Sushi or Raw Cheese?

Not surprisingly, pregnant mothers fear listeria. It can cause miscarriages, premature delivery, and even infant death. A heartbreaking 22% of pregnant mothers who contract listeriosis experience stillbirth.[8]

The most common food-borne culprits hiding listeria bacteria are deli meats, hot dogs, soft cheeses, raw meats, and even raw vegetables and fruits.

Because of this, mothers are told to avoid eating *anything* raw during their pregnancies. Salads or fruits are considered lower risk, assuming that you've adequately washed them. But almost every pregnant mother knows she shouldn't eat that sushi!

If you're a lover of some of the more delectable raw animal foods like a soft, raw Brie or a plate of Japanese sashimi, you may find this disheartening.

When I was pregnant, I craved sushi. For my first pregnancy, I religiously stuck to my doctor's advice and avoided it. My husband I would go on sushi dates, and I'd eat a tempura (fried) roll made with cooked imitation crab, or smoked salmon. There was never any chance that the food I was eating was raw. In my second pregnancy, I told my midwife I wanted sushi and she told me to indulge! After all, raw seafood is some of the most nutrient-dense animal food on the planet, not to mention a sacred food for fertility and pregnancy in almost all traditional cultures.

At first, I grappled with the idea. What if something happened? The guilt would crush me. Then again, if something happened, I'd feel guilty no matter how "perfect" I'd been. If you're playing the blame game, there's always something to blame yourself for, isn't there?

Then I realized that pregnant women routinely eat sushi in Japan. If they had a sweeping epidemic of listeria because of this habit, surely eating sushi would be taboo there, too?

I decided to set my limits. Since I didn't really know what went into the safe handling of raw, sushi-grade fish, I decided not to eat sushi I prepared at home. I'd only eat fresh sushi from a source I trusted, a source with an impeccable kitchen that would answer my questions.

After taking such reasonable precautions, I indulged.

It felt amazing. My body was craving it, and I gave it what it wanted with a clean conscience.

My general philosophy regarding foodborne illness risk is this: Know your farmer. Look them in the eye. Go to their farm and see the living conditions of their animals. Ask questions. I'm serious. Most farmers are quite proud of what they do, and they love telling you about where they source their feed or how they rotate pastures.

Why does knowing your farmer reduce your risk? Well, for one thing, you're dealing with them person to person. Unless they're a scoundrel or sociopath, that actually means something to them. They value you. They see your pregnant belly, and wouldn't want to put you unnecessarily in harm's way. Unlike a behemoth corporate machine that's faceless and impersonal, they actually have the capacity to care. That care makes them careful.

Plus, a smaller, pasture-based operation is simply far less likely to be riddled with pathogens. There's too much sunshine, space, and health to be a breeding ground for disease. It's what gave rise to the old farmer's adage, "The sun is nature's disinfectant." When asked about the relative safety of pastured-poultry operations in the wake of a nationwide egg recall for salmonella, Joel Salatin said,

> "So far, not one case of foodborne pathogens has been reported among the thousands of pastured poultry producers, many of whom have voluntarily had their birds analyzed. Routinely, these home-dressed birds, which have not been treated with chlorine to disinfect them, show numbers far below industry comparisons. At Polyface, we even tested our manure and found that it contained no salmonella.
>
> Pastured poultry farms exhibit trademark lush pastures and healthy chickens with deep-colored egg yolks and fat. As with any movement, some practitioners are excellent and others are charlatans. Knowing your product by putting as much attention on food sourcing as you do on planning your next vacation is the way to insure accountability."[9]

Once you know your farmer, weigh the risks. I ate raw egg yolks from pastured hens routinely during all three of my pregnancies with no fear of salmonella. Even among conventional battery hen eggs, the risk of contracting salmonella is one in 10,000. From pastured hens? The risk is almost non-existent.

On the other hand, I didn't eat raw soft cheeses. Soft cheeses run one of the largest listeria risks even among the cleanest of cheese making facilities.

The risk greatly diminishes as the cheese ages, so I heartily pampered myself with aged raw *hard* cheeses like Gruyere or cheddar from grass fed cows instead.

See, I can be reasonable.

Will a Glass of Red Wine Really Harm My Baby?

Fetal Alcohol Syndrome is the result of heavy drinking during pregnancy. Because of this, all alcohol sold in the U.S. now sports labels warning pregnant women of the dangers of consuming alcohol.

However, many midwives recommend moms drink a glass of red wine to relax, particularly during the third trimester. Furthermore, in many European countries, light to moderate consumption of alcohol during pregnancy is considered normal and even healthy. So, who is right? Why is the advice so conflicting?

Until recently, there has never been a study measuring the effects of light or even moderate drinking during pregnancy. The studies only addressed heavy drinking—defined as "five drinks or more per day"—or no drinking at all. That's because the risk isn't really coming from women who like to have a beer with their husbands after work or a celebratory glass of champagne on New Year's. Rather, it's coming from women who don't restrict their heavy alcohol intake at all, and the studies on heavy drinking are meant to convince them of the permanent damage they're doing both to their child and to themselves when they continue to drink that way.

Then, in 2010, a large study on light drinking during pregnancy was published in the *Journal of Epidemiology and Community Health*. It studied 11,513 children whose mothers reported on their drinking habits while pregnant. The study followed the mothers through their pregnancy, birth, and the first five years of the child's life. For the purpose of the study, "light drinking" was defined as two units of alcohol no more than once or twice per week, when a standard unit is 7.9 grams—approximately one small glass of wine. The British research found no negative effects—at all—of such light drinking on five year olds. In fact, the children were slightly less likely to have behavioral problems and performed somewhat better on cognitive tests than children whose mothers had abstained.[10]

In 2012, a series of five Danish studies were published in the *British Journal of Obstetrics and Gynecology*. They also monitored alcohol consumption in pregnant mothers and studied the children of those mothers again at age five. These studies defined low consumption as one to four drinks per week

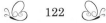

and moderate consumption as five to eight drinks per week. Heavy consumption was nine or more per week, and binge drinking was defined as having more than five drinks in a single sitting on any single occasion. A drink is defined as 12 grams of alcohol.

Not only did this series of studies find no negative cognitive, emotional, or neurological effects in the children of light to moderate drinkers, but it also found no harm to children from binge drinking![11] Heavy drinking, of course, resulted in the typical and well known alcohol side effects—behavioral problems, lower attention spans, learning disabilities, etc.

So, what do these studies mean for you? Where should you draw the line?

With my first pregnancy, I did everything by the book. I had not been a social drinker before getting pregnant, so "giving up" alcohol for my pregnancy didn't feel like a sacrifice at all. Yet after the birth of my son, I purposefully acquired a taste for red wine so that I would no longer be oddly left out at social gatherings.

It had an unexpected side effect. I loved it. The dry, yet full-bodied flavors delighted my taste buds. My taut neck muscles unwound. My shoulders relaxed. I could easily smile and put the stresses of the day behind me. While I still didn't drink daily, I did grow attached to my quiet nighttime ritual of curling up with a good book in one hand and a glass of Australian Shiraz in the other.

So, when my second pregnancy came, I finally had to confront how I felt about drinking when expecting. I knew that some cultures embraced light drinking. I'd heard rumors of the Irish and their Guinness, the French and their wine. Surely if their children were all turning out with fetal alcohol syndrome, the culture would make drinking while pregnant a taboo, wouldn't they?

I applied a little common sense. Since the baby growing in me was being nourished by my blood, I figured that it wasn't so much about *how much* I drank, but my *blood alcohol levels*. No, I didn't walk around with a breathalyzer, but I did gauge my own body's response. Feeling a little lightheaded or tipsy would be going too far, I decided.

In the end, I had almost nothing to drink during the first trimester, and perhaps an average of 1 tall glass of red wine every two or three weeks for the rest of that pregnancy. I opted to follow the same standard with my third baby, too. These children were both born plump at full term, have nice wide dental arches and straight teeth, good vision, and rarely, if ever, get sick. And my placentas? My midwives practically wrote sonnets to those babies.

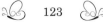

I know what I chose isn't right for everyone. Each of us has to draw our own lines in the sand, question our own comfort levels. Ultimately, I decided to put my trust—yet again—in traditional cultures.

We've been purposefully brewing alcoholic beverages for at least 10,000 years.[12] The ancients knew of both the benefits of light consumption, as well as the risks of excess. Some of the oldest Ayurvedic texts we have called it a "medicine" if drunk in moderation and a "poison" if abused.[13] And red wine? We've been making it pretty much the same way for at least 8,000 years.[14] There is no question in my mind that low levels of alcohol can contribute to health and wellness. How many studies do we need showing that red wine is rich in antioxidants? Or that those who drink wine in moderation have a lower risk of catching a cold?

At real issue here is the fact that just because something is "safe," doesn't mean it's optimal. We know that babies born to heavy drinkers have altered facial structures. Does that mean that drinking even a small amount can negate the positive effects of your fertility and pregnancy diet? Would your baby's face be that much narrower, leading to dental crowding and the need for eyeglasses in a few short years?

I don't have these answers, and there's been little to no research done on this subject. I do know that whatever small risk I may have passed on to my last two children was *worth* the stolen moments of quiet relaxation I enjoyed while pregnant with them. At the time, my midwife had argued that it was more dangerous for me to be stressed out than it was to have a glass of red wine. Maybe she was right? Maybe a different mother would be stronger than I am, more ascetic. Maybe she would have found different, but equally satisfying ways to relax. Maybe she could eat her pregnancy diet and rigidly avoid every potentially harmful substance known to man, including alcohol. Maybe, you're her.

Chapter 8

Beyond Nutrition:
Exploring Alternative Treatments for Fertility & Pregnancy

Our society is enamored with science. Unless we can scientifically prove a claim, we doubt it. Seeing that, it's not hard to understand why we place so much emphasis on what those with scientific authority say—like our doctors.

Yet our doctors are trained to treat sickness and medical emergencies, not health. So, why do we turn to them for advice about how to be healthy? Furthermore, our primary care doctors are not medical researchers. They only know what they were taught in medical school, what drug company sales representatives claim in literature and training sessions, and what they read in the latest professional journals (assuming they keep current with the latest professional journals).

We know enough about marketing to question the information provided by drug company sales representatives. There is no way that a salesman's information is going to be unbiased. Yet, we still put a lot of stock in the scientific research that goes into reports published in medical journals.

Have you ever stopped to ask yourself who funds the research that gets written up in medical journals? Most of these studies are either funded by the drug industry directly, or indirectly funded by the drug industry through universities (which receive their funding from the drug industry).

I am not writing this to knock down the medical profession. If I'm in a car accident, I want to be taken to the nearest emergency room and treated. I want a paramedic on the scene to check me out and give first aid. If I've got an acute illness, I want a doctor to diagnose it and prescribe the antibiotic that best treats it.

That said, I don't want to turn to a medical doctor for help if more natural treatments can return me to health more quickly.

In this chapter, we're going to explore some of these alternatives to standard medical practice—particularly those that can be helpful for fertility and pregnancy.

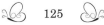

Why Seek Out Alternatives?

According to the *Journal of the American Medical Association*, 106,000 people die each year from taking properly prescribed drugs according to directions in the United States.[1] These are known as "adverse drug reactions," and are commonly accepted risks associated with taking medicinal drugs.

However, adverse drug reactions are only a small part of iatrogenic deaths in the United States (iatrogenic deaths are deaths induced inadvertently by a physician or surgeon or by medical treatment or diagnostic procedures). The table below indicates the total number of iatrogenic deaths by all causes in the U.S.

Total Iatrogenic Deaths in The U.S.

Condition	Deaths
Adverse Drug Reactions	106,000 [2]
Medical error	98,000 [3]
Bedsores	115,000 [4]
Infection	88,000 [5]
Malnutrition	108,800 [6]
Outpatients	199,000 [7]
Unnecessary Procedures	37,136 [8]
Surgery-Related	32,000 [9]
TOTAL	783, 936

In 2009, heart disease claimed 599,413 lives. It was the leading cause of death in the United States that year, according to CDC reports.[10] Too bad the CDC didn't do what I just did and combine all iatrogenic deaths into a single lump sum. Then they could report the truth. Our medical industry unintentionally kills more people each year than heart disease does.

Yet despite these statistics, most of us still trust the medical industry to take care of us. We trust them to tell us what to eat, what pills to take, and what procedures to undergo. Did you know that on average, a medical doctor in the U.S. only receives 23.9 hours of instruction in nutrition during their entire eight years in med school? Some medical schools offer as little as two hours. Two hours![11]

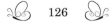

Modern medicine shines when treating acute conditions. We've mastered the art of cleaning and suturing wounds in a sterile environment. We've learned how to help bones knit together well, give people new hearts, and combat many infectious diseases.

But the most frequently treated health issues are not acute. They're chronic. A 2011 survey of primary care providers revealed that nineteen out of the top twenty-five reasons patients seek medical care are for chronic disease symptom management.[12] These are the same chronic diseases, mind you, that are notoriously absent from cultures who've never embraced the modern foods created by industry.[13]

Our medical system is just not set up to focus on nutritional or alternative therapies for healing, particularly for healing and reversing chronic conditions. It's beyond the scope of most doctor's expertise.

Again, I don't want to berate doctors. I've got nothing against them. But you can hopefully start to understand why a growing number of people are opting for alternative care. According to a study sponsored by the Centers for Disease Control, 49.8% of adults in the U.S. opted for some form of alternative health care in 2002.[14] This is up from 42.1% in 1997, so it's likely that the numbers are even higher today.[15]

Maybe you're already a believer. You've visited an acupuncturist or chiropractor and experienced relief. You bought that homeopathic cold remedy or sought to boost your immune system with nutritional supplements when you felt the telltale tickle in the back of your throat, warning you of an impending sinus infection.

Maybe you're not a believer. It doesn't change the fact that more and more patients are taking matters into their own hands and seeking out alternative solutions.

In 1997, Americans spent more than $27 billion on these therapies, exceeding out-of-pocket spending for hospitalizations. They also went on more patient visits to alternative medicine practitioners than they did to their own primary care physicians.[16]

Why are people so eager to seek out alternative therapies? The crux of the issue is that people would have no reason to seek out alternative medical options if modern medicine was solving their health-related difficulties.

Perhaps that's why so many are turning to alternative fertility treatments as well. A recent survey published in the journal *Fertility and Sterility* found that nearly one third of the surveyed couples sought help from acupuncture, herbal therapy, and chiropractic care. Participants were 85% more likely to try the alternative treatment if conventional in-vitro fertilization attempts had failed.[17]

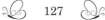

Acupuncture for Fertility

Acupuncture, in conjunction with herbal treatments, has been the primary form of Chinese medicine for at least 4000 years. Although it is popular in the U.S., it has not been extensively studied here. Because it involves the insertion of thin needles in the skin, it makes it difficult to design experiments that adequately control for placebo effects. And unlike most new pharmaceutical drugs in the pipeline, it lacks a well-moneyed backer willing to pour billions of dollars into research to prove its effectiveness.

That said, however, there *is* evidence that acupuncture can be helpful for couples trying to conceive. A 2002 German study measured the results of acupuncture treatments done in conjunction with IVF treatments. The study found that when acupuncture preceded the IVF treatments, the combination was 62.5% more successful in inducing pregnancy.[18] It is important to note that the acupuncture treatments used in this study weren't even the typical course prescribed by traditional practitioners for increasing fertility, but were rather one-time treatments administered immediately before embryo transfer to see if they could make the transfer more successful. And—wonder of wonders—they did!

A recent meta-analysis affirmed these positive results when looking at the results from seven different trials.[19] To my knowledge, no study on the full course of traditional acupuncture fertility treatments has been done.

But what is acupuncture? And how could it possibly increase fertility?

According to classical Chinese medical theory, we have channels of energy running through our bodies. You can liken them to rivers. The paths they take bring nourishing energy to the various tissues and organs. If these pathways are blocked or slowed down by some kind of physical or emotional stressor, they become stagnant. The parts of your body that are no longer receiving a steady stream of this life energy suffer, and the disruption presents itself as pain, discomfort, or disease—including infertility. Acupuncture affects these energy channels by pressing ultra-fine needles into specific points to help stimulate the energy pathways so that they can unclog and flow in a balanced way.

Given that there's no way to measure or quantify these energy pathways in Western science, people here have sought out alternative theories to explain how acupuncture works.

According to traditional Chinese theory, there's an acupuncture point on your little toe that is along the same energy meridian as your eye. So, if you have eye troubles, they'll stimulate the point on your little toe. In a research study at the University of California at Irvine, researchers used MRIs to look at the brain while patients received acupuncture treatment. When the little toe was activated, the part of the brain that regulates vision lit up![20]

What explains this phenomenon?

There are a couple of theories, but perhaps the one that holds the most weight to a Western mind is called the *nerve-reflex theory.*

All of your organs and tissues are surrounded by your autonomic nervous system. It's the visceral nervous system, controlling all the involuntary actions of your organs—the things our body does just to keep going, but without our conscious control (like your heartbeat, digestion, etc.). This system constantly sends information about your physical condition to your brain. If your internal organs have any kind of disorder, these information impulses create a reflex response on the surface of your body. In scientific jargon, it's known as the *viscerocutaneous reflex.* It's why you may sometimes have a sensitive spot on your skin, spasms, inexplicably tight muscles, an oily patch of skin, itchiness, pain, or even redness and other discoloration. The most well-known example of this is when people experience pain in their right surface abdominal muscles when their appendix is inflamed. Often the reflex response is near the injured organ or tissues, but many times it is far removed—as with your eyes and your little toe. Regardless, the correspondence is there.

According to the nerve-reflex theory, acupuncture works by harnessing these channels in the other direction. You stimulate a spot on the surface, and it sends a nerve signal along the reflex pathway to the organs or tissues associated with that spot. The tiny little incision created by the needle—too small to cause pain or actual injury—is just enough of a signal to get your nervous system to pay attention to the organs or tissues linked by the autonomic reflex response. This can increase blood flow and bioelectrical impulses, thereby helping those organs and tissues heal themselves or simply function more efficiently and optimally.

However acupuncture works, many have been impressed by how well it does.

This led Dr. Robert Chang, a prominent fertility specialist at Weill Cornell Medical College, to publish a report suggesting that acupuncture might improve a woman's chances of conceiving because it's relaxing, it can help regulate reproductive hormones, and it can even improve the lining of the uterus, where the embryo needs to be implanted before it can develop.[21]

While I've never personally used acupuncture, I don't find these ideas unreasonable. Plus, I'm encouraged by firsthand accounts from women,

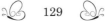

such as Jackie Apuzzo, who sought help from talented and established acupuncturists.

In 2002, *The Los Angeles Times* featured Jackie in an article on acupuncture. They shared that after "nine years of unsuccessful efforts to have a baby, including failed in vitro fertilization, a miscarriage and a diagnosis of endometriosis, the 37-year-old social worker finally visited an acupuncturist on the advice of a friend. After two months of acupuncture treatments and a regimen of Chinese herbs, she became pregnant."[22]

Likewise, Lucy Appert, a 36-year-old mom, suffered through five years of heartrending fertility problems because of a rare pregnancy liver dysfunction that wouldn't let her carry a baby to term. She endured two miscarriages and a stillbirth at eight and a half months. She was at the end of her rope when she decided to try acupuncture treatments. Two months later, she conceived. She continued to see her acupuncturist throughout her pregnancy, and credits the therapy for enabling her to give birth to Henry. "It really was a miracle," the new mom gushed to reporters. "It's one of these weird things that Western medicine can't explain."[23]

If you think you want to experiment with acupuncture therapy, I recommend asking around to find a well-respected acupuncturist, who has had much success helping patients overcome their health complaints. It's important to be selective because acupuncture is a traditional medical art that requires a lot of training—and a fair amount of natural ability—to master. If you want good results, shop around for the best practitioner you can find.

Chiropractic Care for Fertility and Pregnancy

I bet if you asked ten of your friends if they'd ever been to a chiropractor, at least one person would say they had. I wouldn't make the same bet for acupuncture therapy.

That's because chiropractic care—at least for back and neck pain due to injuries—is widely accepted among Westerners. Got rear-ended by a lady who was talking on her cell phone and not paying enough attention to the road? Her car insurance company will likely cover thousands of dollars' worth of chiropractor care. Fall off your ladder while hanging Christmas lights? Your health insurance coverage will likely pay for you to have anywhere from ten to twenty chiropractic adjustments to prevent future injury or complications.

In general, chiropractors are concerned with the diagnosis, treatment, and prevention of disorders in the neuromusculoskeletal system. Most of what they do involves manipulating your spine and other joints with their hands, although many integrate other therapeutic modalities as well. What's less widely accepted is the belief that chiropractic spinal alignments can do more than just remove back pain. I know I hadn't ever considered the possibility until one day when a friend of mine told me about something crazy insane that she'd done for her five-year-old son.

You see, at three years old, he'd been perfectly potty trained. Then his baby sister arrived on the scene and he started having "accidents" in his pants. My friend had assumed it was all part of some psychological need to get attention, and had treated it like a disciplinary issue.

But nothing helped. After a couple years, she sought medical help for her son's growing incontinence. Doctors said there was little they could do. Hopefully, he'd grow out of it.

At the recommendation of a friend, she took her son to a highly sought out local chiropractor. He did a single adjustment on the boy, and his incontinence was cured.

"But how?" I asked. I'd never known chiropractic care could do anything at all like that.

"Well, apparently he had a vertebra just slightly misaligned in his spine at the exact spot that sends signals to us to let us know to go poop. He wasn't willfully pooping in his pants at all. He just didn't feel the urge like the rest of us do."

"WOW. I mean, wow!"

Yes, I turn monosyllabic when I'm dumbfounded.

A few months later, her son wrestled with some other boys and got seriously knocked around. No injuries, but the incontinence returned—this time in his bladder. He'd just pee. Mortified and embarrassed, he tried to hide it. But he couldn't do that for very long.

Another trip to the chiropractor's office, and he was fixed up right as rain.

Now, tell me, does this make sense to you? Can you believe this story? I'm not lying. I've got no reason to. My friend certainly wasn't lying either.

If you can believe this story, then you can probably also see why chiropractic care can help with fertility struggles.

Basic chiropractic theory goes something like this. If your spinal column is even slightly misaligned, you are compressing vital nerves that help your body's organs function properly. If these nerves can't properly signal these organs, then those organs fail to function optimally. Sometimes, that suboptimal functioning is obvious, as in the case of my friend's incontinent boy. Other times, you may not really notice. Instead, you just have organs

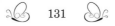

not working as efficiently as they could. Maybe this expresses itself as you getting slightly sicker then your co-workers, or you always struggling with constipation despite eating the best of diets. If you have a spinal misalignment in the area that sends nerve signals out to your ovaries, then you may experience a hormonal imbalance significant enough to affect your fertility.

That's what happened to Karen Bulch, a 44-year-old who had unsuccessfully been trying to get pregnant for four and half years. Fertility doctors had told her she was simply too old, that she had about a 5% chance of ever getting pregnant again. So, she'd given up. On her first visit to the chiropractor, he noticed a subluxation—or slight misalignment of the vertebrae—in Karen's lower back. He warned her that when the spinal column got realigned, the restored nerve flow might return her ability to become fertile. She didn't really believe in the possibility, but tucked away the memory of his words to her as a nice thought. A month after her first visit, she was pregnant. Dr. Kimes, her chiropractor wasn't surprised. "I've been in practice for 12 years and I've seen it happen with many women," he said.[24]

Karen isn't alone. According to a 2003 study published in the *Journal of Vertebral Subluxation Research*, fourteen out of fifteen infertile women conceived after receiving enough chiropractic treatment to correct spinal misalignment (anywhere from three to twenty months of treatment, depending on how severe the misalignment was). In the study, spinal realignment helped a woman who had been without a period for twenty years start menstruating again. It also caused one woman's PCOS to heal.[25]

Do I believe chiropractic care is a panacea for curing fertility problems? No. But it can be another tool in your tool belt, and it may just come in handy.

Even mothers-to-be who don't struggle with fertility enjoy chiropractic care during their pregnancies. It can help keep your spinal column aligned to ensure that neural pathways to your uterus and placenta aren't blocked. It can help with back and hip pain. It can even help ensure your baby's in the best possible position for birth.

Imagine that you're pregnant. Imagine that your doctor or midwife just told you that your baby is not yet in the head down position. Delivering feet first? Most doctors won't touch that vaginal birth with a ten-foot pole, opting instead for a C-section. Your heart races. The blood drains from your face. You try to keep listening to your birth professional's reassurance that all will be well, that your baby is still perfectly happy and comfortable inside you. Will your baby turn on her own? Will your doctor have to turn the baby? Does your doctor even *do* that? Is that even considered safe anymore?

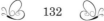

Even if your pregnancy is otherwise low-risk, a baby presenting abnormally near the end of the term almost always results in a surgical birth. In 2003, 87.2% of all breech babies were born by C-section.[26]

That doesn't mean your doctor won't try turning the baby. It's even got a medical name—*external cephalic version*. It involves pushing on the baby through your abdomen. It's highly uncomfortable and can cause a host of complications including vaginal bleeding, premature rupture of membranes, fetal distress and premature labor. Most doctors will shy away from doing this unless you have a very low-risk pregnancy. It's far more likely that your doctor will take a wait-and-see approach.

Maybe your baby will spontaneously turn.

Maybe she won't.

But how did your baby get this way in the first place? Remember that your baby and your body are hardwired to do exactly the right things at exactly the right times to bring this baby into the world whole and healthy. It's the same hard-wiring that has them latching on to your breast within minutes of birth, even though they've never nursed before. So what's the problem? Nicole Whitehead, a doctor of chiropractic care in Mooresville, NC who specializes in treating pregnant mothers, infants, and children, had this to say:

"Something is preventing the natural process from occurring in your situation. In some cases, it can be a structural issue within the womb, such as a fibroid or other space occupying presence. Often, pre-term labor is accompanied by abnormal presentation because the 'time to turn' in the baby's programming had not yet occurred. However, according to Danforth's *Obstetrics and Gynecology*, there is no apparent cause for the failure to go vertex over 50% of the time. It would be ludicrous to assume that over 50% of the fetuses in abnormal position simply 'didn't get the memo' about turning head-down. So, it logically follows that something is preventing the baby from turning."[27]

Back in the 1970s, a chiropractor named Larry Webster noticed the link between misaligned sacral or pelvic bones and babies that presented feet first. This led him to create a series of gentle adjustments—now known as the *Webster Technique*—to re-align the pelvic region of pregnant women. He used this technique on more than a thousand pregnant mothers. In 90 percent of cases, the babies turned to the correct, head down position within just three adjustments.[28]

How did it work? Why was it so gentle and safe compared to the practice of *external cephalic version* tried by doctors?

Look at any anatomy textbook, and you'll likely see your answer. Your uterus is attached to your pelvis and sacrum by ligaments on all sides. When you're pregnant, your body produces a hormone called relaxin. Relaxin's job is like its name implies. It's meant to relax your soft tissues to make it easy for your organs, ligaments, and other musculature to realign to make room inside you for a growing baby. It also makes it easy for your sacrum and pelvic bones to become misaligned. If that happens, the ligaments holding your uterus in place pull against each other awkwardly, twisting your uterine muscles just enough that it constrains the baby, trapping the baby in whatever position it was in at the time the muscles became torqued. By using the Webster Technique, a chiropractor can realign your sacrum and pelvic bones, releasing the abnormal pull on your uterus and freeing your baby to do what she's hardwired to do—turn to a head-down position.

It also has another side effect. The properly aligned pelvis and sacrum widens your birth canal, too. And what does that spell? An easier birth.

Natural Remedies During Pregnancy

One of the first things you'll get when you visit a birth practitioner after you get pregnant is a list of over-the-counter medicines (and sometimes foods) to avoid. These medicines are things many people rely on to treat common colds, allergies, aches or pains, insomnia or other minor ailments.

If you're one of those people who immediately reach for the Tylenol when you have a headache or the Sudafed when you start feeling congested, then you may be wondering how you're supposed to cope with these symptoms if they show up when you're pregnant.

Do you just suffer through them? Do you stumble into your office with red eyes and a scratchy throat? Take more sick days? Turn down the lights and drink more water when your head is pounding?

If herbal supplements or other natural remedies are new to you, consider this your introduction. I wrote this section for you. Please bear in mind that I'm not a medical doctor, licensed nutritionist, herbal practitioner, or any kind of health professional. I'm a mom who's been pregnant three times, and this is how I found my relief.

If you're looking for something more comprehensive and covering just about every imaginable complaint that needs alleviating, I highly recommend the book *Wise Woman Herbal for the Childbearing Year* by Susun S. Weed. That lady knows her stuff!

Allergies, Coughs, Sore Throats, & Colds

It is no secret that pregnancy hormones cause your mucus membranes to swell. This helps keep your cervix healthy, but the thicker mucus also makes it far easier for a minor sinus irritation to turn into a full-blown infection. So, how should you treat respiratory congestion when you first notice it?

~ *Neti Pot*

The first and easiest line of defense is a neti pot. Neti pots are traditional to eastern cultures and have been used for thousands of years to clear out nasal passageways naturally. To use a neti pot, you simply fill it with warm, slightly salty water. You then pour the saline water into one nostril and let it drain out the other. After a complete pot of water is used on the first nostril, blow your nose and repeat the process for the other nostril. If you are not yet sick or suffering from allergies, doing this once per day can clear out any irritants that might cause an inflammatory response from your sinuses. If you have noticed sinus drainage or congestion, then you can use the neti pot as many times per day as you need to in order to find relief. During my worst days of congestion, this is usually about once every 3 to 4 hours.

~ *Acerola Powder*

Acerola is naturally high in vitamin C. When you first start noticing symptoms of encroaching illness (that telltale tickle in the back of your throat), you can start treating yourself with 8,000 milligrams of vitamin C per day for up to three days. Take enough acerola to confer 1,000 milligrams of vitamin C every one to two hours while waking. I once read in a physician's newsletter that this little protocol prevented 80% of all colds and seasonal allergy bouts in his patients. Studies done on vitamin C dosing in relation to colds have only tested significantly lower doses—only up to 200 milligrams per day. But even at that low level, the consensus of studies show it can reduce the duration of the cold, if not the symptoms.[29]

~ *Echinacea*

Echinacea taken three times daily in the following amounts have been shown to decrease lengths of colds and flu:

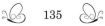

- Dried root (or as tea)—0.5 to 1 gram;
- Freeze dried plant, 325—650 milligrams;
- Tincture (1:5)—2-4 milliliters.

~ *Licorice*

Licorice root tea is extremely helpful in reducing sore throat pain. If the sore throat is accompanied with a cough, try to find an herbal tea or tonic that contains licorice root in addition to other common herbal cough remedies (like elder berries, cinnamon, spikenard root, and wild cherry).

~ *Apple Cider Vinegar*

Mix three tablespoons of apple cider vinegar with three tablespoons of honey, then add a few ounces of hot water. Sip on this tonic for sore throats. ACV kills 100% of all streptococcus bacteria on contact, so it's very helpful in preventing lingering sore throats and strep throat.

Anemia

As you found out in the last chapter, most cases of "anemia" during pregnancy aren't really anemia. Rather, it's simply the body struggling to keep up with a dramatically increased blood volume. Aside from eating iron-rich foods and taking the organic iron supplements (like Floradix or Ferrofood) mentioned in Chapter 7, you can also help your body naturally absorb more of the iron you eat with the following herbal remedy:

~ *Yellow Dock*

Take one to two dropper squirts of the liquid tonic one to three times per day, depending on the severity of your symptoms. Yellow dock has the added benefit of enhancing liver function which translates into: less nausea, constipation relief, and a better immune response, among other things.

Cramps

Muscle cramping, particularly at night or right upon waking is most often a result of a magnesium or calcium deficiency. If you are not getting enough calcium in your diet, try to increase the amount of grass-fed dairy you are eating each day. If you cannot tolerate dairy, add more bone broths to your diet. If your diet is high in dairy products and calcium and you still

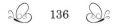

experience these cramps, it is almost certainly a magnesium deficiency. Try supplementing externally with magnesium oil, or internally with enough natural magnesium to get an extra 400-500 milligrams per day.

~ Salt

While correcting the above dietary imbalances will prevent future cramping, a pretty sure fire way to immediately relieve your cramping is by putting a pinch of real salt under your tongue in combination with stretching & massaging the cramped muscles. If your cramp is in your legs or feet, pull the foot towards your body instead of pointing toes downward.

Headaches

There are two kinds of headaches: migraine (or vascular) headaches characterized by throbbing, sharp pain and tension headaches character-ized by steady, constant, dull pain.

~ Magnesium

Magnesium deficiency is a known cause of both types of head-aches. If recurring headaches are a problem, it's wise to try supple-menting with magnesium first. The most effective way to absorb mag-nesium is transdermally, so applying external magnesium oil is often the best way to get extra magnesium.

~ Ginger

Ginger is a known anti-inflammatory and has been used for thou-sands of years in traditional Chinese medicine to eliminate head-aches. The recommended amount is one or two 500-600 milligram capsules taken with water up to four times per day.

~ Tiger Balm (White)

This is a mix of traditional Chinese herbs set in a minty-camphor base, but unlike many Chinese remedies it's available on the mass market at most major drug stores. To relieve tension headaches, just dab a little of it on your temples and close your eyes while relaxing for ten to fifteen minutes. It works wonders!

Heartburn

Heartburn is caused by the lower esophageal sphincter muscles relaxing enough to allow stomach acids to spurt up into the esophagus. Unfortunate-

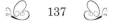

ly, pregnancy hormones tend to relax muscles in the body (including your sphincter muscles), so heartburn is more likely to occur.

~ Marshmallow Root

When combined with water, marshmallow root swells to form a soft, soothing, protective gel. This provides heartburn relief within about fifteen to thirty minutes. Take two capsules after meals.

Insomnia

Stress during pregnancy seems to be magnified. Small things become much harder to cope with, and mothers-to-be often find themselves unable to sleep despite being very tired.

~ Valerian Root

Many scientific studies have verified that valerian root is as effective (if not more so) as small doses of benzodiazepines in helping people fall asleep. Thankfully, unlike the pharmaceutical drug, it's also perfectly safe for pregnant women. It also has no residual morning "hangover" so that women can wake well-rested. Take 30 minutes before bedtime: one to two grams of the dried root, four to six milligrams of tincture, or one to two milligrams of fluid extract.

~ Relaxing Sleep Tonic by Herb Pharm

This herbal tonic mixes valerian root with other, complimentary, safe herbs for a well-rounded sleep tonic. Take one to two dropper squirts approximately 30 minutes before bed.

Natural Childbirth Options

If you're trying your best to eat healthy, whole, "sacred" foods to build natural fertility and have a healthy pregnancy, you're avoiding hormones, antibiotics, and other medical drugs whenever possible. Why would it be wrong to take these drugs when pregnant, but suddenly safe to take them in labor?

In the United States, nearly every woman gives birth in a hospital. I myself had a very positive experience giving birth to my first child in a hospital in Ashland, OR. It was completely natural and intervention free. My newly born son stayed in the room with me instead of being carted away to a nursery, and a lactation consultant on staff at the hospital helped get me started

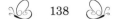

breastfeeding with aplomb. But my hospital? It was rare. It had been certi-fied by the World Health Organization to be both baby and mommy friend-ly. That basically means they did everything possible to encourage natural births, reduce C-section rates, and facilitate mother-baby bonding.

In the U.S., birth is considered a medical event, so much so that you can't get new insurance coverage while pregnant without paying premium prices for your "pre-existing condition." Yet despite the thousands of dollars we pour into each birth, despite the fact that the vast majority of births happen in hospitals with doctors present and emergency staff on call, despite all of this—we have comparably horrible birth outcomes.

Birth outcomes are measured by incidences of death and illness during labor, birth, and the period of time shortly after birth. We're told we have some of the best medical care in the world. Maybe we do. But in 2011, we were ranked forty-ninth in the world for infant mortality.[30] That means that there are forty-eight other countries where it's safer for your baby for you to give birth than here in the United States. We were ranked 121st in maternal mortality.[31]

I'd like to propose that these appalling statistics might be because we're mistreating birth. The countries with the best birth outcomes are those that don't treat birth like a medical event. Instead, women's prenatal and birth care are handled by trained midwives, and OBGYN's are consulted only in actual medical emergencies or abnormal cases.

One of my friends had her baby the typical way—in a hospital where she eventually received an epidural and pitocin when her contractions slowed. She couldn't stop praising the epidural and was so, so thankful to be out of pain. Her exact words? "I would rather take a gun to my own head than ex-perience birth without an epidural."

While that is probably an exaggeration, it expresses a common senti-ment. Birth is painful. Epidurals are safe, medically-approved ways to re-lieve that pain. Therefore, it MUST be the way to go!

But did you know that birth without pain is possible—without the use of epidurals or other drugs? I should know. My first birth was completely pain-free and all-natural.

When I say that, people often think I'm exaggerating or even lying. I'm not.

Not long ago, women giving birth were routinely knocked out with chlo-roform, strapped into tables on their back, and had babies extracted with forceps and vacuum suction. This was considered a humane practice, for it saved women from the pain of childbirth.

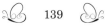

Then one obstetrician named Grantly Dick-Read saw the unthinkable—a completely intervention-free, natural birth where the mother gave birth in peace, quiet, and with a smile on her face. He had been taught that such births were impossible, so he set out to study natural childbirth. In 1944, he published his findings in a book that changed history—*Childbirth Without Fear.*

In his book, he identified what he called the Fear-Tension-Pain Cycle. The basic idea is this: When women are afraid of birth, it increases the tension in their bodies, and this in turn increases the pain they experience in labor. It's a cycle because the more pain the woman experiences, the more she is afraid, and so forth.

The key to a pain-free, all-natural birth is breaking this cycle. Instead of Fear-Tension-Pain, women can experience Faith-Relaxation-Pleasure.

Many natural childbirth methods arise from trying to break the cycle through relaxation techniques meant to help ease tension. But if you still have underlying fear, relaxation becomes increasingly difficult as birth progresses. *The most effective natural childbirth techniques are those that help you eliminate fear at its root, as well as keep you relaxed.*

It's no wonder that most women fear giving birth. Every television show and movie that's shown us a birth depicts women screaming, insulting their husbands, or being rushed into operating rooms. No one shows that it can be pleasurable, peaceful even.

Given all this, birth educator Laura Shanley concludes:

"Eliminating fear is not impossible, for there is something that is much more powerful than the most all-consuming fear—FAITH. Faith is believing that all is well . . . Faith is trusting that our bodies were designed to give birth safely and painlessly. Faith is accepting the fact that we are the creators of our lives and our births. Faith is not the opposite of reason. Having faith does not mean that we sit back and do nothing during our pregnancy. When we have faith, we understand the psychological origins for the majority of pain and problems most women encounter in labor and we do our best to face and conquer our fears. We don't run to "specialists" for "blood work" or urine tests or vitamins, for we know that with good food (neither too much, nor too little), fresh air, exercise, and the proper beliefs, our babies will thrive."[32]

But how can you re-program your subconscious? How can you root out your fear? There are many faith-based approaches that seek to eliminate the fears associated with birth—some even tailored to religious faiths. Personally, I used and recommend *hypnobirthing* (think: hypnosis meets birth).

When people think of hypnosis, they think of a practitioner hypnotizing away someone's will so that they quack like a duck or flap their arms. It's bizarre, slightly unbelievable, and foreign.

Yet truth be told, we've all been self-hypnotized before. Have you ever gotten in your car when you had a lot on your mind? Suddenly you're at a familiar destination, and you don't really remember the drive you took to get there? You were completely safe, obeyed all the traffic rules, avoided speeding or collisions, and navigated the roads between Point A and Point B with ease. And yet, your mind was so occupied with your thoughts that a part of you wasn't, in fact, paying attention to the road at all. That's self-hypnosis. It's allowing your mind and body to do one thing well—like drive to a familiar destination—while simultaneously keeping your mind very focused on a series of involving thoughts.

Hypnobirthing is a method of birthing that allows you to enter into self-hypnosis during childbirth. Moms who want to use hypnobirthing are encouraged to take classes offered by a trained hypnobirthing practitioner early on in their pregnancy (at say, four or five months). During the classes, they'll learn how to self-hypnotize, and then they're set free to practice it for an additional four or five months on their own. The more you practice the self-hypnosis routines, the more second nature it becomes (much like the everyday commute between work and home). Eventually, you can reach the point where a single trigger word can do in seconds what originally took you eight minutes of following a self-hypnosis script to accomplish.

Hypnobirthing seeks to completely eliminate fear during childbirth, while simultaneously keeping the mother fully relaxed. If the baby presents normally, this results in pain-free, often quick deliveries. There are several different hypnobirthing methods out there (Hypnobirthing: The Mongan Method, Hypnobabies, etc.). They all do basically the same thing, but utilize different scripts at various stages of pregnancy and birth.

To my mind, hypnobirthing is the epitome of natural childbirth options because it roots out fear, replacing it with faith in positive affirmations. It also helps the body fully relax and self-anesthetize so that relaxation and pleasure result. However, that's not to say it's the only worthwhile technique. (It's just my favorite!) There are other natural childbirth methods out there, and I encourage you to explore them.

Chapter 9

Breastfeeding and Homemade Formulas

After the birth of my first child, someone asked what being a mom was like.

"Soggy," I replied. Tears of stress. Tears of joy. Baby burp-ups dribbling down my back—at least until I had an epiphany and understood why mothers of infants never lack burp cloths. Baby poops erupting out of diapers onto onesies. Breast milk leaking through nursing pads and drenching my shirts. (I eventually just opted to go topless when no one else was around. Seriously.) In the words of Nina Planck, "Very soggy indeed."[1]

And nursing? No one ever told me that it could take up to thirty minutes a session for a newborn! You know how many times a day a newborn is supposed to nurse, on average? Eight to twelve. I spent six hours a day nursing. Talk about a life-altering experience.

I was not only a mother. I was a milk-machine. Thankfully, I never experienced any major issues with nursing my three little ones that a quick internet search on some breastfeeding forums couldn't help me figure out. My first two children nursed until about two and half. My third one still latches on regularly at twenty-one months.

None of my children have ever been fed commercial formula. I guess I'm lucky that way.

Infant formulas have a long history. After all, if a mother was unable to nurse and a wet nurse could not be employed, babies had to be given *something* for food. The first commercially available infant formulas came on the market at the turn of the last century, but even as late as 1950 only about half of all babies raised in the U.S. were ever fed any kind of infant formulas.

Then came the marketers. Rather than marketing to mothers, they hit upon a new strategy. They began to market their formulas to doctors and hospitals. Within a decade, the tide had turned. By 1970, 75% of all babies raised in the U.S. were being fed infant formulas.[2]

At roughly the same time, a resurgence in breastfeeding also began. Mothers began advocating for breastfeeding as more nutritious, healthier, and better for infants.

Now, thanks to the research and campaigning of organizations such as the World Health Organization, the Centers for Disease Control, and the

U.S. Department of Health, most moms acknowledge that "breast is best." And according to data released by the CDC in 2010, roughly 75% of all babies in the U.S. are breastfed for at least some part of their infancy. Forty-four percent of all babies are still being breastfed at six months of age, and 24% are still being breastfed by the time they reach a year old.[3]

Yet, the number of babies being fed formula has not decreased. Rather, what the numbers indicate is that moms are attempting to breastfeed, but failing.

Only 35% of all babies are exclusively breastfed at three months of age. By six months old, the numbers drop to a paltry 15%. In other words, moms begin breastfeeding with the best of intentions, but soon end up supplementing with formula.[4]

What does this mean? Is breastfeeding really so hard? How can something that mothers have done for generation after generation, for thousands upon thousands of years, be so difficult?

I'm sure a hefty percentage of the numbers have to do with convenience. Despite being told that "breast is best," we're also told that formula is a reasonable alternative. We were all raised on formula and turned out fine. Didn't we?

So, when faced with returning to work, taking trips or vacations away from our babies, or any other choice that would make exclusive breastfeeding near impossible, we happily pick out a commercial infant formula to supplement our breast milk.

But from my own talks with breastfeeding mommas, I'm confident that most mothers start supplementing because they feel that breastfeeding is "too hard." Their supply was low. Their baby preferred bottles, but pumping enough to keep up with the baby's demand was impractical. They experienced pain or tenderness when nursing and got quickly discouraged.

In this chapter, we'll cover the basics on how to feed your newborn, and hopefully we'll keep those discouraging thoughts at bay by empowering you with knowledge.

Is Breast Always Best?

Thankfully, this is one thing that doctors, nurses, researchers, the scientific community, history, and natural moms agree on: breastfeeding has a myriad of benefits.

Babies who breastfeed have greater natural immunity, catch fewer infections, are less likely to die from SIDS (sudden infant death syndrome), are less obese, suffer from fewer allergies, are less likely to get asthma, and have higher cognitive development.

Moms who breastfeed experience a regular infusion of a cocktail of love-enhancing hormones to help them bond with the baby, delay fertility an average of twelve months if following a nurse-on-demand model, and have a reduced risk for cancer, arthritis, and heart disease.

Put simply, enough studies have been done, enough public bias swayed, that no one doubts the benefits of breastfeeding anymore. It's why so many moms start to breastfeed.

Yet most of us were raised in a generation when breastfeeding children was not the norm. Our mothers tried and failed, or didn't try at all. They have very little, if any, advice to pass on to us.

If my nipples suddenly become very sore and itchy, is that normal? What about if my breast becomes tender? Why does my baby sometimes gag or choke when nursing? Uh oh. Why is my baby's poop … green???!!!

Without anyone to guide us, we turn to books, blogs, internet forums, and even professionals. Yes! There is an entire field of work called "lactation consulting," and licensed lactation consultants teach classes, offer demonstrations, run support groups, and help counsel moms one-on-one through their nursing problems.

In my opinion, the scariest place to learn about nursing is the internet. Sure, you can type in a search query and instantly find an answer. But you could also wander into a breastfeeding forum, let drop that you don't co-sleep, and be labeled the devil incarnate because you *dare* to put your newborn to sleep in a different room from yours!

Or, you could be reading a blog about breastfeeding, comment with a bit about how you've had to wean your eight-month-old daughter because she went on a two week long nursing strike, and quickly be berated by an angry horde because you "gave up" on nursing "without even trying!"

These are called Mommy Wars. And they've infected the internet like flies on poop. Zealous moms do research, become impassioned advocates for a particular way of doing things, then insist that it is absolutely right for all parents, all mothers, all kids, everywhere, and for all time. When moms with opposing views get together in the same online space—watch out!

In the middle of the Mommy Wars, it's not uncommon to read someone rabidly profess that breast milk is always best. No matter what you eat, they say, your breast milk will be *perfect*. Your body will always make the most amazing milk possible, even at your own expense. It will prioritize nourishing and protecting that baby.

This—there's no other way to put it—is bunk. Pure myth.

It goes against all common sense.

We know that the composition of breast milk is always changing due to the mother's environment and diet.[5] The more nutrient-dense the mother's diet, the more nutrient-dense the mother's milk. We also know that the opposite is true—the less nutrient-dense the mother's diet, the less nutrient-dense her milk.

How many news stories do we need to see before we believe it? In 2011, a Russian mother was charged and found guilty of killing her baby with alcohol poisoned breast milk.[6] She'd been binge drinking, nursed her baby while she was wildly drunk, and her baby died. It's utterly tragic, but it's also common sense. We know that what you eat and drink changes your milk. It's why we tell moms to practice common sense when drinking and nursing. Want a beer? That's okay. Just drink it after you put your baby to bed at night, don't drink to excess, and wait a few hours for the alcohol to leave your system before you nurse your baby.[7] (Be warned that alcohol actually reduces milk supply, so you shouldn't indulge if you have any supply issues.)

Earlier in 2011, a vegan mother was charged with criminal neglect after her exclusively breastfed infant died of nutrient-deficiencies common to vegans—lack of vitamins B12 and A.[8] Clearly, her nutrient-poor diet made nutrient-poor breast milk. And her baby, her little bundle of joy, died.

We can't keep perpetuating this myth.

Is breast universally, always, unequivocally best? I think it's clear that in some cases, the answer is obviously no.

This should give us pause. It is not enough to simply breastfeed your baby. Your own diet matters!

The good news here is that if you're eating the diet described in Chapter 6, you're pretty much going to have the most nutrient-dense breast milk on the planet.

Breastfeeding Basics

If breastfeeding looks easy when you see other, more experienced mothers do it, that's because it is. But it may not *come* easily. Your baby may have a poor latch. Your nipples may get sore. Your baby may sleep too long and just neglect to nurse. Your baby may prefer a bottle. Some of these things can be prevented. Others can only be corrected. But, they'll all work out in the end.

That's because breastfeeding is natural. It's how babies have *always* been fed. So, begin with a boost of confidence, Momma. You. Will. Succeed.

The single most important thing we've "re-discovered" about breastfeeding since it's resurgence on the popular scene is that *you make milk in response to your baby sucking at the breast*. Like economics, it's all supply and demand. The more demand your baby presents—the more milk your baby actually removes from the breast, the more you'll make.

With that in mind, this is how you'll get off to a fantastic start:

- **Breastfeed early**. As soon as your baby's born, put him to the breast. In an ideal scenario, you'd be nursing mere minutes after giving birth to your baby. Breastfeeding releases the hormone oxytocin—the hormone necessary for uterine contractions. The sooner you can get your uterus contracting again, the sooner you'll safely birth your placenta without any hemorrhaging.

- **Breastfeed often**. Really, anytime your baby is awake, it's a good time to offer your breast. Newborns can nurse between 8 and 12 times a day. And, since it's all about supply and demand, the more the merrier.

- **Don't allow caregivers to give your baby a bottle or a pacifier**. Until nursing is well-established, you don't want your baby learning to like any nipple better than yours. It can encourage him to have the wrong kind of latch (a suck from a bottle uses a different tongue motion and muscle pattern than a suck from a real nipple). Plus, bottles often have an easier flow; babies don't have to work as hard to get milk from a bottle. This can make them prefer the bottle to your breast. And, what does that spell? Decreased demand. And that means....? Decreased supply! Good. You're getting it!

- **Nurse on demand**. Healthy babies develop their own feeding schedules. Follow your baby's cues for when he's hungry, and give him what he wants. Typical cues are stirring, rooting, and putting those tiny little hands in their mouths. At least until nursing's established (and arguably even a while after that), your breast is the best pacifier! When at the breast, allow your baby to nurse as long as he wants—as long as he's actively nursing. Then, offer the other breast. It's simple, and no clocks are necessary.

Don't over think it.

Geesh. I've read a lot of breastfeeding literature in my day. Half of it seems like it was written by people who don't want you to breastfeed your baby. They make it sound so complicated.

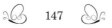

Don't lean this way or that; you'll hurt your back. Don't let the baby nurse at this angle; it'll hurt your nipples. Don't position your baby like that; position him like this.

The truth is, breastfeeding happens. Your baby is born with the need to suckle. As soon as he's anywhere near your breast, he'll start rooting around, nuzzling his adorable little head into your breast, smacking his lips open and closed. If you put your baby's open mouth anywhere near your nipple, it's a done deal. He'll latch on.

The only trick is to try to get a "good" latch. It'll be more efficient for your little one, and it will cause you less pain.

Here's the typical rulebook for getting a good latch:

- Tickle the baby's lips to encourage him to open wide. With your baby's mouth wide open, pull him close so that the chin and lower jaw moves into your breast first.

- Aim to get his lower lip as far away from the base of your nipple as possible, so that when he latches down he'll get a large mouthful of breast.

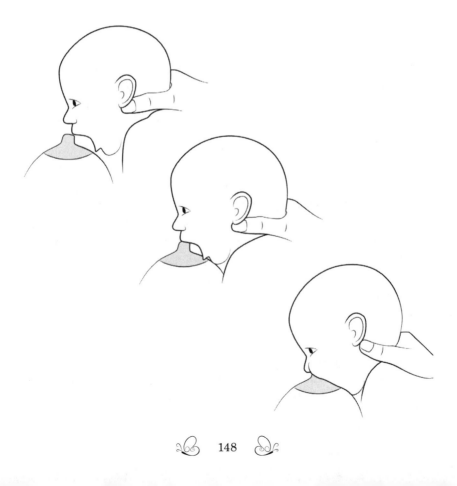

Hopefully, it will look something like this:

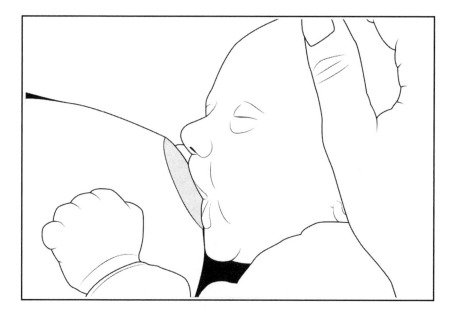

But, even if it doesn't, the most important thing is that the latch feels comfortable without any hurting, or pinching. I also like to make sure that the baby's lips are turned out, like little fish lips. If they're not, just slide your finger in between his lips and your areola and gently turn them out. Hold your baby in a way that supports his head, ideally so that his head doesn't have to turn while nursing.

Some babies are born lazy. Their latches are poor. Their suck is weak. They like to sleep all the time. It may take time for you to get your baby to latch on well. If so, that's okay. Just remember to be patient and give both you and the baby a break. If you start to stress too much, spend time cuddling skin to skin with your baby held upright between your breasts, rocking him or singing. If your baby wants to suck, but your nipple is off limits because of stress or discomfort, offer your pinky instead. Try to breastfeed again when you're not so stressed.

Try different positions.

With my first son, breastfeeding was so new to me, I didn't want to "mess up." I found a position that worked—the typical "cradle hold" on a breast-feeding pillow—and stuck with it. When my boy woke up in the middle of the night to nurse, I'd whip out my U-shaped breastfeeding pillow, sit up cross-legged in the bed, and nurse him in the cradle hold. This, despite the fact that he slept an arm's reach away in a bassinet on level with my mattress.

With my second son, I used the same bassinet positioned against my bed again. But this time when I had to nurse him, I just rolled over, picked up my son, and rolled back. I nursed him laying down, even from his earliest days. It was magical! A revelation! I could actually get real rest while breastfeeding in the middle of the night.

Don't be intimidated by different holds. Try them out. They may be useful in unforeseen ways.

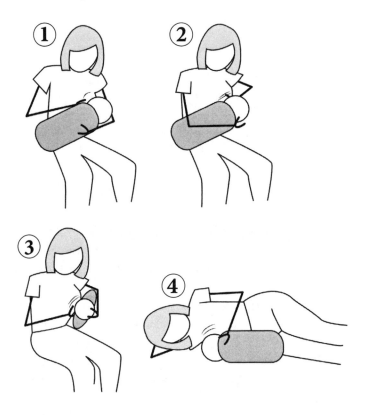

#1—The Cradle Hold: This is the hold we all revert to. It's easy. It's comfortable.

#2—The Cross Cradle Hold: This is useful for babies that have a weak suck, or babies that are on the small side. It gives extra head support and may help babies stay latched

#3—The Football Hold: If you've had a C-section, have large breasts, or have

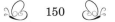

an over-active milk letdown (more on that in the troubleshooting section), this may be the hold for you!

#4—Lying Down: This is also good for mommas post C-section, but especially wondrous for those of us who need to get extra rest while nursing.

Don't despair! Troubleshoot

Forceful Let-down and Oversupply

If your baby experiences any of the following symptoms, you may have an overactive let-down (meaning that your milk comes out too fast, or in too great a quantity):

- gagging, gasping, or coughing while nursing as though milk is coming too fast
- pulling off the breast while nursing
- spitting up often, or being gassy
- poop has a green tint

Decrease your supply by implementing block nursing. This is when you nurse the baby on one breast exclusively for a certain block of time. Start with 2-3 hours and increase in half-hour increments if needed. *Do not restrict nursing at all*, but any time that baby needs to nurse simply keep putting baby back to the same side during that time period.

Is Your Milk Supply Low?

You already know that supply is all about demand—empty those breasts of milk frequently, and your body will make more milk to fill them back up. You probably won't have any problem establishing a nursing relationship. Most moms don't.

But eventually, something changes. Maybe your little one starts making fewer dirty diapers, or starts demanding to nurse more frequently—a lot more frequently. Before you get scared that something's off or wrong, know this: Your nursing relationship will *always* be evolving and changing. Just when you think something is "normal," your baby will spontaneously start doing something different.

If you feel insecure about whether or not your baby is getting enough milk, all you have to do is make sure your little one is gaining weight. *If your baby is gaining weight well on breast milk alone, then you do not have a problem with milk supply, period.*

But, what if you're not quite sure about your baby's current weight gain? So long as your baby is making enough wet and dirty diapers (which given today's disposable diaper technology can be as few as 4-6 diapers per day) then consider these changes normal, and not a sign of a low milk supply:

- *Your baby nurses frequently.* Some people are full of terrible advice. They tell you that you shouldn't nurse your baby more frequently than every 4 hours, but your girl likes to nurse every hour or two. News-flash! Breast milk is digested quickly—more quickly than formula—so breastfed babies need to eat more often than formula-fed babies. Or maybe your baby just likes to suck. Nursing is about more than just food. Or maybe your baby just wants the comfort of being near you.

- *Your baby suddenly increases the frequency and/or length of nursings.* This is most likely a *growth spurt*. They only last for a few days, a week at most. Don't offer your baby formula when this happens. Instead, just nurse, nurse, nurse. Supplementing will inform your body that the baby doesn't need the extra milk, and your supply will drop.

- *Your baby doesn't nurse as long as she did previously.* Once your baby gets good at nursing, he'll get *really* good at nursing. What used to be a 45 minute nursing session for a newborn becomes a 5 minute session. It's no big deal. Your little guy is just way more efficient than he used to be.

- *Your baby is fussy.* She's a baby. Babies fuss. Is your baby fed? Check. Is her diaper clean? Check. Does she want to be held? Check. Does she want to be swaddled, rocked, put down to sleep? Check. There are a host of things that can make your baby fussy, and sometimes you'll never find the reason.

- *Your baby guzzles down a bottle of formula or expressed milk after nursing.* Many babies will willingly take a bottle even after they have a full feeding at the breast. They do that. Be wary of doing this, though. If you frequently supplement your breast milk with formula, you'll decrease your supply. Remember, it's all about demand.

- *You get very little or no milk when you pump.* Most women can't pump more than a dribble when they start. It's not an accurate measure of your milk supply. Babies are far more efficient than machines at getting milk out of your breast. Trust me.

If your baby is having trouble gaining weight, then it's possible that you have a low milk supply. Remember, it's all about supply and demand. So, put more demand on your breasts to make more milk. Nurse more frequently. Avoid pacifiers and bottles, allowing your baby to comfort nurse at your breast instead. Feed only breast milk (no formula or water). Make sure your little one is nursing efficiently, with a good latch. If you need help, ask for it! Call in a lactation consultant.

Baby Refuses The Breast

Maybe your baby wasn't exposed to your breast, but a bottle first. Or maybe your baby's grown attached to bottle feeding and just doesn't want to nurse. Or maybe your baby bit you one day and you yelped, and now he doesn't want to go back to your breast again. Regardless of the reason, the same strategies for coaxing the baby back to the breast apply.

First, the number one rule is to *feed your baby.* A baby who is not nursing is a baby who *can't* nurse. It's not as if you can starve your baby into desiring the breast. So, this may mean that you supplement by bottle-feeding your baby the homemade formula you'll learn how to make later in this chapter. While supplementing, make sure you keep your own supply up by pumping often and regularly!

To coax your baby back to the breast: make sure the baby has *easy access to your breasts* (spend time with her topless and/or bra-less); offer lots of *skin to skin contact*, particularly just as baby is waking or going to sleep; *offer the breast often,* but *don't pressure the baby* to nurse (pretend their refusal doesn't affect you); *wear your baby* or keep them near you (even when sleeping); and finally, seek out opportunities to *comfort nurse* (offer your breast as a pacifier).

Sore Nipples

There are a number of causes of sore nipples. If your baby is newborn, the first thing to do is to make sure your baby is *latched on properly.* Review the earlier section on getting a good latch for tips.

If your baby has a proper latch, but your nipples are still sore, your baby may be having *sucking difficulties.* This can either be due to a physical impediment (such as tongue-tie) or laziness. Tongue-tie can easily be fixed by a pediatrician, but your baby's laziness may simply have to be outgrown. In the meantime, use the techniques below to help comfort your sore nipples.

You and your baby may also be experiencing *thrush*, a yeast infection probably contracted by the baby during a vaginal birth. Thrush is the kind of infection that you and your baby can pass back and forth. If you think you have thrush, look for the telltale white patches inside your baby's lips and mouth. Natural treatments are available, but first time mommas probably want to go to a doctor to confirm the diagnosis and find out what options are available for treatment.

If only one nipple or breast is sore, you may be experiencing a *plugged duct* or *mastitis*. A plugged duct is a blocked milk duct. You may actually see a blocked nipple pore, or the plug maybe further back in the ductal system. You may notice a hard lump that may feel tender, hot, swollen or look reddened. Mastitis is an infection in your breast, has the same symptoms as a plugged duct, but is usually more intense and accompanied by a fever. The treatment for both is the same. Nurse as frequently as you can. Before nursing, apply a hot compress to the breast and gently massage the area—massages in hot showers work wonders. Loosen bras (or go without) so that you don't in any way restrict milk flow. Nurse on the affected breast first. While your baby's nursing, massage the plugged area. If 24 hours of this treatment bring no improvement, visit your doctor.

You can also experience sore nipples during *hormonal changes* brought on by ovulating, having your period, or being pregnant. Some women find supplementing with magnesium helps prevent nipple soreness due to hormonal changes.

If your baby is older, nipple soreness may be caused by *irritation* caused by teething (extra saliva and an adapting latch), eating solids (baby nursing with remnants of solid foods in their mouth), or a new soap or detergent.

To comfort sore nipples, try the following:

During Nursing:
- Breastfeed from the uninjured (or less injured) side first. Baby will tend to nurse more gently on the second side offered.
- The initial latch-on tends to hurt the worst—a brief application of ice right before latching can help to numb the area.

After Nursing:
- Use a salt water rinse (dilute ½ teaspoon of salt in 1 cup of warm water)

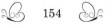

- Apply a medical grade lanolin ointment like Lanisoh (www.lansinoh. com/products/hpa-lanolin) to the nipple
- Keep nipples exposed to air (Go bra-less! If you do wear a bra, be sure to change damp nursing pads immediately.)

Making Homemade Formula

When breastfeeding isn't an option, or a baby's diet must be supplemented, your inner nutritionally-obsessed-self will take one look at the labels on commercial formulas and cringe.

What's wrong with commercial baby formula?

Commercial baby formula is laced with soy proteins, even in the non-soy milk based versions. Did you know that soy contains phytoestrogens—plant-based hormones that mimic estrogen in our bodies?[9] That's why babies fed soy formula have blood levels of estrogen at 13,000 - 22,000 times greater than those who are breastfed or given a milk-based formula.[10] Infants fed commercial baby formula are consuming the equivalent of four birth control pills worth of estrogen daily.[11]

Furthermore, commercial baby formula is full of other industrial by-products. Recent news stories have reported shocking discoveries of everything from arsenic to BPA to rocket fuel in commercial formulas, even in the so-called organic versions. MSG hides in the form of autolyzed or hydrolyzed proteins or extracts.[12] Plus, formulas are iron-fortified (a true danger to young infants) and full of synthetic vitamins and minerals.[13][14]

In general, if you can avoid feeding your infant commercial formulas, you should!

But what on earth are you supposed to feed your baby instead?

I've known quite a few mothers who have made homemade formula using the recipes formulated by the Weston A. Price Foundation. These formulas were specifically designed to mimic the nutrient content of breast milk—and without resorting to industrial foods, byproducts, or synthetic ingredients.

As much as we may want to breastfeed, sometimes we just can't. Life gets in the way. Maybe you had breast reduction surgery, or maybe pumping at work is turning out to be far more difficult than you'd first imagined. Maybe you had to take a course of prescription drugs for an illness or injury, and you've got no pumped milk on hand to feed your little one in the meantime. Or, maybe you'd like your husband to feed your baby, and the idea of pump-

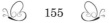

ing makes you shudder. Maybe you're not a mother at all, but a single dad trying to do the best for his infant child. Whatever the reason, aren't you glad that there are better alternatives than commercial formula?

These homemade formulas are a bit complicated at first. You'll want to measure each ingredient precisely and follow the instructions *exactly*. Any changes can alter the content and availability of the nutrients, and that may harm your baby. But eventually, making them will become second nature. You'll be able to whip them together in fifteen minutes and have enough formula on hand to last you a few days.

In an emergency, when the ingredients for homemade formula aren't on hand, the Weston A. Price Foundation recommends fortifying 1 cup of the commercial formula with a soft-boiled egg yolk and half a teaspoon of fermented cod liver oil.

Homemade Formula Recipes
 (from the Weston A. Price Foundation)

Raw Milk Baby Formula
Makes 36 ounces.

Our milk-based formula takes account of the fact that human milk is richer in whey, lactose, vitamin C, niacin, and long-chain polyunsaturated fatty acids compared to cow's milk but leaner in casein (milk protein). The addition of gelatin to cow's milk formula will make it more digestible for the infant. Use only truly cold-expressed oils in the formula recipes, otherwise they may lack vitamin E.

The ideal milk for baby, if he cannot be breastfed, is clean, whole raw milk from old-fashioned cows that feed on green pastures and are certified free of disease. For sources of good quality milk, see www.realmilk.com or contact a local chapter of the Weston A. Price Foundation.

If the only choice available to you is commercial milk, choose whole milk, preferably organic and unhomogenized, and culture it with a piima or kefir culture to restore enzymes.

<u>Ingredients</u>
- 2 cups whole raw cow's milk, preferably from pasture-fed cows
- ¼ cup homemade liquid whey (See recipe for whey, below) Note: Do NOT use powdered whey or whey from making cheese (which will cause the formula to curdle). Use only homemade whey made from yoghurt, kefir or separated raw milk.

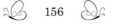

- 4 tablespoons lactose[1]
- ¼ teaspoon bifidobacterium infantis
- 2 or more tablespoons good quality cream (preferably not ultra-pasteurized), more if you are using milk from Holstein cows
- ½ teaspoon unflavored high-vitamin or high-vitamin-fermented cod liver oil or 1 teaspoon regular cod liver oil[2]
- ¼ teaspoon high-vitamin butter oil (optional)[1]
- 1 teaspoon expeller-expressed sunflower oil[1]
- 1 teaspoon extra virgin olive oil[1]
- 2 teaspoons coconut oil[1]
- 2 teaspoons Frontier brand nutritional yeast flakes[1]
- 2 teaspoons gelatin[1]
- 1-⅞ cups filtered water
- ¼ teaspoon acerola powder[1]

1. Available from Radiant Life 888-593-8333, www.radiantlifecatalog.com.

2. Use only brands of cod liver oil that are naturally-made and free of synthetic vitamins.

Instructions
- Put 2 cups filtered water into a pyrex measuring pitcher and remove 2 tablespoons (that will give you 1-⅞ cups water).
- Pour about half of the water into a pan and place on a medium flame.
- Add the gelatin and lactose to the pan and let dissolve, stirring occasionally.
- When the gelatin and lactose are dissolved, remove from heat and add the remaining water to cool the mixture.
- Stir in the coconut oil and optional high-vitamin butter oil and stir until melted.
- Meanwhile, place remaining ingredients into a blender.
- Add the water mixture and blend about three seconds.
- Place in glass bottles or a glass jar and refrigerate.

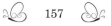

- Before giving to baby, warm bottles by placing in hot water or a bottle warmer. NEVER warm bottles in a microwave oven.

Variation: Goat Milk Formula

Although goat milk is rich in fat, it must be used with caution in infant feeding as it lacks folic acid and is low in vitamin B12, both of which are essential to the growth and development of the infant. Inclusion of nutritional yeast to provide folic acid is essential. If you're going to use it in the Milk-based formula above, please compensate for goat milk's low levels of vitamin B12 by adding two teaspoons *organic raw chicken liver, frozen for fourteen days, finely grated* to the batch of formula. Be sure to begin egg-yolk feeding at four months.

Liver-Based Formula

Makes about 36 ounces.

Our liver-based formula also mimics the nutrient profile of mother's milk. It is extremely important to include coconut oil in this formula since it is the only ingredient that provides the special medium-chain saturated fats found in mother's milk. As with the milk-based formula, all oils should be truly cold-expressed.

<u>Ingredients:</u>

- 3¾ cups homemade beef or chicken broth
- 2 ounces organic liver, cut into small pieces
- 5 tablespoons lactose[1]
- ¼ teaspoon bifidobacterium infantis
- ¼ cup homemade liquid whey (See recipe for whey, below)
- 1 tablespoon coconut oil[1]
- ½ teaspoon unflavored high-vitamin or high-vitamin fermented cod liver oil or 1 teaspoon regular cod liver oil[2]
- 1 teaspoon unrefined sunflower oil[1]
- 2 teaspoons extra virgin olive oil[1]
- ¼ teaspoon acerola powder[1]

1. Available from Radiant Life, 888-593-8333, www.radiantlifecatalog.com.

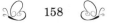

2. Use only brands of cod liver oil that are naturally-made and free of synthetic vitamins like Green Pasture's Blue Ice Fermented Cod Liver Oil (www.greenpasture.org/public/Products/CodLiverOil/index.cfm), Garden of Life's Olde World Icelandic Cod Liver Oil (www.gardenoflife.com/Products-for-Life/Foundational-Nutrition/Olde-World-Icelandic.aspx), or Corganic's Raw Cod Liver Oil (www.rawcodliveroil.com/where-to-buy/).

Instructions:

- Simmer liver gently in broth until the meat is cooked through.
- Liquefy using a handheld blender or in a food processor.
- When the liver broth has cooled, stir in remaining ingredients.
- Store in a very clean glass or stainless steel container.
- To serve, stir formula well and pour six to eight ounces in a very clean glass bottle.
- Attach a clean nipple and set in a pan of simmering water until formula is warm but not hot to the touch, shake well and feed to baby. (Never heat formula in a microwave oven!)

Chapter 10

Baby's First Foods

Ages ago, I visited a WIC nutritionist. WIC is the U.S. governmental supplemental nutrition program for Women, Infants, and Children. They provide mothers and mothers-to-be with vouchers that can be used on specific food items at participating grocery stores. They also offer educational services, including consultations with nutritionists.

I don't remember much of what my WIC nutritionist told me, but I do remember this. She recommended that I start introducing solid foods to my baby at four months old.

"Begin with an infant cereal, like rice cereal," she said. "Just mix a little bit in with their milk in a bottle or sippy cup. At about six months, you can start introducing the solid baby foods you buy at the supermarket."

This is standard nutritional advice for infants in the U.S.

If you walk down the baby food aisle of your grocery store, you'll notice a couple of things. The first is that the food is often segregated and marketed according to age. First you'll find your infant formulas, followed quickly by infant cereals. Eventually you reach a section of "teething" snacks like cookies and crackers. Then, finally, shelves loaded with cooked, flavorless, mashed vegetables, fruits, and meats. Meats take up the tiniest section. Snack foods, fruits, and sweet vegetables like sweet potatoes and peas take up the lion's share of space.

If you fed your baby according to how the baby food is marketed, your baby's first solid food would be infant cereals. Then, when your baby started teething at somewhere between four to eight months old, you'd start feeding them crackers and cookies meant to soothe their gums. At roughly the same time, you'd start introducing them to mashed sweet fruits and vegetables. Only later would you feed them pureed meats, eventually "graduating" into lumpy meats.

As much as I hate to say it, this whole marketing scheme is backwards. It's almost the exact opposite of how successful, traditional cultures introduced foods to their babies. Cereal grains as a baby's first solid food? It's practically unheard of—barring times of famine or war. In the cultures that do traditionally introduce grains first, it's usually been fermented into a gruel and served with other nutrient-rich foods like tuna or fish roe.[1]

Taking a look at some of the historically common first baby foods can teach us a few things.

In Oceania, a tribe called the Yafar pre-chew fish, grubs, and liver for their babies. What do you notice first about that list? The animal foods, or the fact that parents fed babies pre-chewed foods? I can't imagine wanting to feed my baby headless grubs, but I also didn't grow up in Oceania. Pre-chewing food, on the other hand, is an all too common practice around the world. It shows up in many different cultures. Besides mashing the food, pre-chewing also helps to pre-digest the food with enzymes present in our saliva.

If we head to more tropical climates, like Polynesia, we'll see babies being fed *poipoi*—a mixture of breadfruit and coconut cream that has a pudding like texture. Beside human breast milk, coconut is nature's best-known source for lauric acid. It's also rich in the saturated fat your baby's growing brain needs. I find it fascinating that mommas in Polynesia introduced their babies to foods that mimic the nutrient profile of breast milk.

Travel to the Arctic, and you'll see the Inuit feeding their little ones seaweed, seal blubber, and stewed caribou. As with the Polynesians, we see a pairing of animal fats and cooked plant food. Could this be because so many important vitamin precursors found in plant foods, like the beta-carotene in seaweed and breadfruit, need these fats to convert to their true forms in our bodies?

In Mexico, babies are fed egg yolks, *atole* (a fermented corn porridge), and bone marrow soup. The Maori of New Zealand feed babies cooked bone marrow, watercress, fish eggs, crayfish, and seaweed. The Japanese offer a gruel of fermented white rice with fish, fish eggs, and mashed pumpkin.

And what about traditional baby feeding in Western cuisine? How did my European ancestors start feeding their babies solids? Babies usually began eating egg yolks and liver with roasted bone marrow. Vegetables were cooked soft in bone broth before both the veggies and the broth were served to infants.

Compare these foods with the rice and oat cereals, creamed wheat, and grain-based snacks and crackers you find on any baby food aisle here in the U.S. Our modern diet of first foods for babies looks mighty empty, void of nutrients.

But beyond *what* traditional cultures first feed babies, I'm also impressed by *how* they fed them. In almost all cases, babies in traditional cultures eat socially. They're eating right alongside their parents and siblings, at the "family table." And, these solid foods aren't displacing their breastfeeding. On the contrary, the average mother breastfed until her baby was two and half years old. Some cultures nurse far longer, others less. Some tandem nurse a three

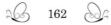

year old and an infant at the same time.[2] My point? Clearly mommas in traditional cultures kept breastfeeding well past the successful introduction of solid foods.

My own grandmother pulled me aside once when she saw me nursing my fourteen-month-old son.

"You're still nursing him?" she hissed at me. "You nurse until your baby has teeth. Then you stop. They can eat after that; they don't need to nurse."

If I had told her that the American Academy of Pediatrics recommends mothers breastfeed for at least a year, then as long after that as is "mutually agreeable" to both mother and child, I don't think she would have blinked.

And the World Health Organization? They're not so forgiving. They encourage mothers to breastfeed for at least two years. Two years! My grandma would have either had a heart attack, or launched into a rant questioning what the World Health Organization knows anyway.

I don't really know what her opinion would have been on baby-led solids. I never had the chance to ask.

Let Your Baby Lead

Baby-led solids (sometimes called baby-led weaning) is an easy, gratifying, and practical way to introduce solid foods to your baby so that they'll readily embrace their place at the table during family meals. And, it's what I chose to do with all three of my children.

I had seen the kids who ate fish sticks and bananas at the dinner table while their parents sat beside them eating sushi or steak, and I did not want my own children to end up that way. More to the point, *I* didn't want to end up that way. Preparing a separate meal for each member of my family? No thank you.

If you follow the baby-led solids model of introducing foods, you will nip that problem in the bud. That's because you'll never be preparing separate, "special" food for the baby that you, yourself don't eat.

With baby-led solids, there's *no spoon feeding and no purées*. Well, butter my butt and call me a biscuit! I could feed my baby homemade, wholesome, nutrient dense foods without having to do all that work making baby food? Sign me up!

Babies sit with the rest of the family at mealtimes, even from the earliest age. When your little one can safely sit up on her own and reach to grab foods with a pincer grasp, usually around six months old, you let her feed herself. At first, it's all about fingers. Eventually, as she grows more coordi-

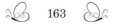

nated, you can give her baby-sized cutlery and let her teach herself how to dig up a spoonful of food and bring it to her mouth. You feed her the food from your own table, plus a few nutrient-rich superfoods.

Babies get to explore various textures, tastes, colors, and smells. They gain confidence and independence. And it turns mealtimes from battlefields into celebrations.

That's because you're not fighting nature. Instead, you're taking advantage of the way babies naturally develop and grow. A baby's digestive system isn't really ready for solids until they are about six months old. It can come earlier for some babies, later for others. But the point is, if you start spoon feeding your baby when she's three months old, you'll never know! You'll miss the developmental and biological cues that your baby is ready to start eating solids.

And just how do you know they're ready? When they ask for it! Your baby will be able to sit up, pick up food, put it in his mouth, and chew it. He'll be able to feed himself, and he'll *want* to feed himself. He'll see you enjoying your supper, and he'll reach for your food. He'll start grabbing at the food on your plate—or the food in your hand.

What does this mean, really? It means no battles. No sitting frustrated next to your baby's highchair, making airplane noises while periodically looking down at your watch. No hassle cooking and pureeing vegetables and meats. No slogging through endless nights of your baby's interminable constipation, gas, or general digestive discomfort. It means trusting in your child's natural inquisitiveness, fascination, and joy.

"But won't my baby choke?" Doctors have long instructed parents to introduce finger foods at around 6 months. This is no different. You're just skipping the spoon-feeding.

Tips for introducing solids

1) Make sure you're offering foods you and your family are already enjoying and eating. Your baby will see you relishing your foods and anticipate doing the same. They love to mimic you, to be like you. If you're taking pleasure in your food, chances are they will, too.

2) Keep offering foods your baby initially doesn't like. Babies will often reject a food one day, then gobble it up another. Sometimes, they'll spurn a food a dozen times before trying it and loving it. If they're rejecting a sacred, nutrient-rich food you really want them to like, try cooking it different ways. For example, if they're rejecting liver, you could offer Liver & Onions (p. 194), Chicken Liver Paté (p. 193), or even Homemade Braunschweiger (p 195).

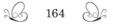

3) Be prepared for the mess. Babies love exploring food, putting it in their mouth, spitting it out, flinging it away. They're not misbehaving. They're learning. Anticipate the mess by putting a towel, rug, or mat underneath their highchair. Or, time the messiest meals to happen right before bath time. This way, you won't have to stress.

4) Relax. Your baby may go days without eating very much at all. You're still breastfeeding, aren't you? It doesn't really matter if your baby eats a lot of solids or not. Just when you think they'll never eat, they'll suddenly develop an appetite again and try new foods with abandon.

In the 1920s, a pediatrician named Clara Davis conducted an experiment that might not fly well today. She offered babies between the ages of seven and nine months old a choice of thirty-three real foods on a daily basis and recorded what they ate.

"With no refined foods to muck up their palates, these children demonstrated an innate wisdom to self-select the foods that met their nutritional needs to create vibrant health, which was monitored by extensive testing. Food selections were not always pretty. One day a child ate seven eggs, while another opted for a handful of salt. Some children ate more fruits, yet others gravitated to the meats. A child with poor bone structure was partial to cod liver oil one hundred thirteen times, on his own accord. While each day's meal did not provide a perfect 'balance,' over the long haul, their nutritional profile conformed to just what they needed."[3]

While thirty-three foods is probably a bit too much for your own attempts, the lesson is clear. Offer variety. Offer nutrient-density. And your baby will choose the right foods at the right time.

Ditch the Infant Cereals

What's wrong with infant cereal?
So glad you asked! First, it's not traditional.
In my nutritional philosophy, tradition has weight. After all, we've survived anywhere from 7,000 to 77,000 generations on this planet (depending

on whose science you believe). If we didn't know how to adequately nourish our children all that time, how did we even get here?

And guess what? Traditional cultures didn't (and don't) feed their young babies infant cereal. Among the few cultures that fed their babies a gruel of grains, their practice radically differed from what we do today. They would either pre-chew the gruel for their babies until they were at least a year old, or the gruel was mildly fermented by soaking the grains for 24 hours or more.

Babies can't digest it fully

In order to digest grains, your body needs to make use of an enzyme called amylase. Amylase is the enzyme responsible for splitting starches. And, guess what? Babies don't make amylase in large enough quantities to digest grains until after they are a year old at the earliest. Sometimes it can take up to two years.

You see, newborns don't produce amylase at all.[4] Salivary amylase makes a small appearance at about six months old,[5] but pancreatic amylase (what you need to actually digest grains) is not produced until molar teeth are fully developed![6] [7] First molars usually don't show up until thirteen to nineteen months old, on average.

Undigested grains can wreak havoc on your baby's intestinal lining. It can throw off the balance of bacteria in their gut and lead to lots of complications as they age including: food allergies, behavioral problems, mood issues, and more.[8]

What does this mean? Don't feed your baby grains (or even highly starchy foods), until all of their first molars have emerged. This means no rice cereals, no Cheerios, no Goldfish, no oatmeal, no infant crackers. It means that when you sit down with them at a restaurant, you shouldn't placate them with the free rolls.

Feeding your baby grains displaces other, more important nutrients

If you feed your baby cereal or other grains, you're doing more than simply sticking them with a potentially indigestible food. You're feeding them an indigestible food in place of something more nutrient-dense. You're feeding them something their body can't really use and starving them of the nutrients they need to grow a healthy brain, nervous system, and bone structure.

What can you feed your baby instead?

It's the million dollar question, and the answer isn't all that hard. It's based on a few key principles.

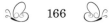

First, babies need fat.

More than 50% of the calories in mother's milk comes from saturated fat. That's for a good reason. Babies need fat in order to grow their brains, nervous system, and cell membranes. The remaining calories come from protein, and carbohydrates in the form of lactose. (And guess what? Newborns actually make lactase, the enzyme necessary to digest lactose. Plus, lactase is also common in raw milk. So, any deficiency in lactase production your baby might have is compensated for by the raw milk you provide them while breastfeeding.) In traditional cultures, it's common to breastfeed children at least two years and generally well into toddlerhood. So, don't fret the saturated fat. In fact, you should embrace it!

Second, babies need lots of the fat-soluble vitamins A, D, & K2.

These vitamins are essential for your baby to grow a strong, sturdy bone structure. They also dramatically affect how your baby's face forms. Remember how our whole goal here is to help our babies develop a wide face with high cheekbones, rather than a narrow face full of crowded teeth, constricted sinuses, and displaced eyes. We've already highlighted the paramount role these fat-soluble vitamins play in fertility and fetal development. They don't stop being vital just because you're baby's been born. We need these nutrients for life.

Again, I trust the wisdom of generation after generation of mothers more than I trust marketers trying to sell me an industrial-waste-product-turned-baby-food. We've got a long history of nourishing our infants well, pre-industrial revolution (the only exceptions being times of famine, war, or poverty).

Let Traditional Wisdom be Your Guide

When it's time to introduce solids, don't buy into the ploy of baby food marketers intent on making a buck. Those are foods that Weston A. Price liked to call the "displacing foods of modern convenience." Rather than opting for convenience, opt for nutrient-density. Give your baby foods that are rich in the kinds of fats and vitamins they need for optimal development.

Age 6-8 Months

- **Broth**—Homemade bone broth is calcium and mineral rich. It's a more nutrient-dense option than water, and not sugar-laden like fruit juice. It also soothes digestion and helps promote an intestinal environment that's hospitable to the "good" kinds of bacteria and yeast that ought to

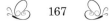

populate our gut. It's a great drink to give to babies when you're feeding them solid foods, and will not cause any adverse reactions like cow's milk or soy milk.

- **Egg Yolks**—Around the world, through the centuries, almost universally, the first solid food we've ever introduced to babies were egg yolks. I recommend the egg yolks from pastured hens.

"Egg yolk supplies cholesterol needed for mental development as well as important sulphur-containing amino acids. Egg yolks from pasture-fed hens or hens raised on flax meal, fish meal or insects are also rich in the omega-3 long-chain fatty acids found in mother's milk but which may be lacking in cow's milk. These fatty acids are essential for the development of the brain. Parents who institute the practice of feeding egg yolk to baby will be rewarded with children who speak and take directions at an early age. The white, which contains difficult-to-digest proteins, should not be given before the age of one year."[9]

You can start introducing egg yolks as soon as your baby shows an interest in eating solid foods. For us, our rule has been that we introduce solids when our babies have been old enough to pick the food up and put it in their own mouth. This usually happens somewhere between 6 to 8 months. I've known mothers who spoon-fed egg yolks to babies at an earlier age (around 4 months). While that's a generally safe practice, it's also work! I like the babies-feeding-themselves model because it's easy.

- **Liver**—Preferably, this is raw, organic liver from grass-fed cows. But even cooked liver has its benefits. You can grate liver that has been frozen for at least 14 days (to kill any pathogens) and mash it into egg yolks to feed it to baby. At this young age, I'd put a scoop of the mix onto a spoon and hand it to baby and let them move the spoon to their mouth. As soon as my babies demonstrated an interest in scooping and spooning their own foods (usually around 10-15 months), I set them loose with their own servings of soft liver patés and braunschweiger. Recipes for both may be found in Part 2 of this book. The Weston A. Price Foundation says this about liver:

"Small amounts of grated, raw organic liver may be added occasionally to the egg yolk after six months. This imitates the practice of African

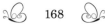

mothers who chew liver before giving it to their infants as their first food. Liver is rich in iron, the one mineral that tends to be low in mother's milk possibly because iron competes with zinc for absorption."[10]

What about liver from industrially raised cattle? While grass-fed is best, followed by certified organic, liver is so nutrient-dense that I don't hesitate to occasionally feed my baby liver from an industrial source. This, of course ignores the ethical issues of feeding ourselves industrially produced animal foods. The truth is that sometimes organic or grass-fed organ meats are hard to come by or afford. So, if you must compromise, you should at least stick to foods that are as nutrient-dense as possible. Because of industrial processing methods, I wouldn't want to feed my baby raw industrial liver products. But I think that if the liver is cooked, eating it is generally preferable to not feeding them liver at all.

If you're worried about industrial toxins being stored in the liver, then I say "Aren't you smart?" Because, of course, that's why you'd prefer organic liver to the alternatives. But, I would also remind you of two things. First, the liver does not store toxins, but helps clean them from the blood so they can be expelled from the body with minimal harm. Second, if you're otherwise doing right by your child's gut (feeding them probiotic rich foods and avoiding sugars & grains), their guts can (generally speaking) handle the elimination of the toxins.

- **Butter**—Again, I'd stick to raw butter from grass-fed cows, but any real butter will do in a pinch. Butter is an easy-to-come-by animal fat, and you should try to stick to feeding your infant foods rich in animal fats as much as possible. You can serve butter on cooked vegetables, or you can simply do what I do and feed it to your baby straight.

Yep, you read right. When we're at a restaurant, instead of placating my little ones with the free rolls, we placate them with the free butter that comes with the rolls!

- **Bananas**—Bananas are one of the few carbohydrate rich foods that are also rich in amylase. So, they come with the enzyme your baby needs to digest them already built-in. You can start feeding your baby bananas when they start making salivary amylase and expressing an interest in eating solid foods.

- **Avocados**—High in quality fats, mild in flavor, and with a smooth texture, many babies enjoy avocados early on.

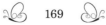

- **Fish Roe**—Tangy, salty, crunchy and juicy, these fabulous first foods are a cornucopia of texture, color, and flavor that almost always delights babies. Plus, they're packed with nutrients like omega-3 fatty acids, B vitamins, vitamin D, and choline—all absolutely essential for a growing brain!

- **Fermented Cod Liver Oil**—½ tsp. per day served (unheated) with food. You may increase the dose as your baby grows, settling finally at 1 tsp. per day when your baby is about a year old.

Age 10 Months

- **Cooked or Stewed Vegetables and Meats**—You can start feeding your baby cooked vegetables and meats when they're old enough to express an interest in these foods and self-feed. I've always enjoyed putting on a small Crock Pot of a bone-broth-based stew featuring meat and veggies and feeding my baby the super-tender foods that come from it over the course of a few days. Cooked fatty fish like salmon, anchovies, and sardines can be introduced now, too.

- **Kefir, Yogurt, and Buttermilk**—These soured milk products are probiotic and help build up a balance of good bacteria in your baby's gut, thus ensuring that they properly digest all their foods. Plus, introducing your baby to the sour taste early can help their palate enjoy more of these nutrient-rich foods later. I'd start by introducing them to just a spoonful or so at a time. As they get older, you can give them more of these foods.

- **Raw Cheeses**—Hard cheeses like cheddar, Gouda, or Gruyere make great snacks and finger foods. Try to get raw cheeses from pasture-fed cows. If raw is not available, give preference to cheeses from pasture-fed cows that haven't been treated with growth hormones or antibiotics.

- **Raw Fruits**—Babies love fruits, and by this age they are sure to be producing enough salivary amylase to break down the naturally occurring sugars in the fruit. Wait to introduce citrus fruits until baby is a year old.

Over 1 Year

- **Raw Milk**—From grass-fed cows, of course. If raw milk is unavailable, try fermenting pasteurized milk from grass-fed cows into kefir, then blending into a runny fruit drink (not as thick as a smoothie).

- **Whole Eggs**—Again, stick with eggs from pastured hens. Soft-boiled, hard-boiled, and scrambled eggs tend to be favorites.

- **Citrus Fruits**—Babies are finally able to digest citrus!

- **Nut Butters**—Nut butters made from soaked & dried or roasted nuts can be introduced.

- **Seafood**—Oysters, clams, scallops, fish roe, shrimp, lobster, crab.

<u>14 -24 Months (or when molars come in)</u>

- **Soaked Oatmeal**—Soak rolled or steel cut oats overnight in equal parts oats to yogurt. In the morning add enough water to reach desired thickness, then boil. Season with plenty of butter and sweeten with a natural sweetener like honey or maple syrup.

- **Sprouted Grains or Sourdough**—If baby digests oatmeal well, branch out into other sprouted grains or sourdoughs.

- **Soaked, Cooked Corn**—If baby digests other traditionally prepared grains well, try introducing corn (that's been soaked in lime).

- **Soaked, Cooked Legumes**—Soak legumes for 18-24 hours in warm water with a dash of Probiotic Whey (p. 177), lemon juice, or vinegar. Rinse well, then cook until tender.

A part of me recoils from listing the average ages above. Why? Because they're averages. The whole point of baby-led solids is that you feed your baby according to his or her developmental cues. Rather than trusting in an average, trust your own parental instincts. You know your baby.

You know if she can sit up, grab food, put it in her mouth, and chew it. You know if her tummy's upset or if she's constipated by something she's eaten. You're the one who changes her poopy diapers and sees whether or not her foods are giving her an allergic rash—that telltale ring of red around her anus is no accident. You know her likes and dislikes, her moods, her patterns. *You're the expert.*

So, use those averages as a guide. Mostly, pay attention to the *order* of when these foods are introduced, as well as their nutrient-density.

You'll do just fine.

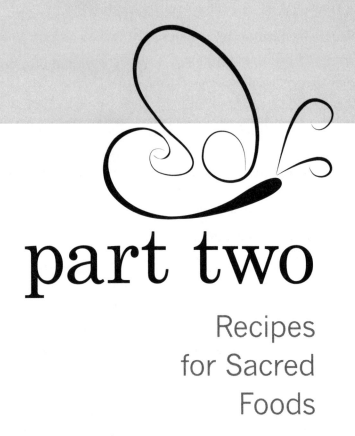

part two

Recipes
for Sacred
Foods

Opting out of the industrial food system means making a lot of food at home so that you know the ingredients were sourced well. It means substituting "good" ingredients for "bad" ones in some of our favorite recipes. Instead of using canola oil, you'll now reach for the olive oil or coconut oil. Instead of using farmed fish, you'll grab a wild-caught fish. Instead of buying supermarket beef from a cow finished on a feedlot, you'll buy a side of grass-fed beef from a local rancher. Instead of cooking your favorite cake with white flour, you'll substitute sprouted flour instead. These sorts of adaptations come easily.

What's really intimidating to most are the sacred foods for fertility, pregnancy, breastfeeding, and nourishing a growing baby. Liver? Who among us cooks that regularly? Fish roe? Clams? Oysters? Scallops? What about adding in the old-fashioned, naturally fermented condiments and beverages that are so essential for our gut health? If your roasted chicken carcass has only ever made its way to the trash, even something as simple as making a homemade bone broth may seem daunting. And eggs! Falling into a rut with eggs can be disastrous if you're trying to eat at least two a day. How are you supposed to eat that many eggs without going crazy with boredom?

Consider this part of the book an aide to helping you prepare and enjoy these sacred foods.

It ought to go without saying that you'll be sourcing all these ingredients well—using the principles in Chapters 4 and 5 as your guiding light. I hope this small collection of recipes gets your creative juices flowing, bringing you one step closer to embracing these sacred foods as a routine part of your diet.

Snacks and Condiments

Odd Bits: Organs & Bones

Seafood

Eggs

Chinese Tomato and Eggs / 203

Grain-Free Apple Pancake Rings / 204

Basil Eggs Ringed in Bell Pepper / 205

Texas Style Crustless Quiche / 206

Eggs Poached in Marinara / 207

Egg Drop Soup / 208

Egg-Stravagant Breakfast Smoothie / 208

Summer Squash Omelet
with Tomato Gravy / 209

Feta Egg Scramble / 210

Tomato Parmesan Egg Cupcakes / 210

Beverages

Fizzy Lemonade / 211

Homemade Orange Soda / 211

Homemade Almond Milk / 212

Homemade Flavored Kombucha / 212

Grain-Free
Apple
Pancake
Rings
p. 204

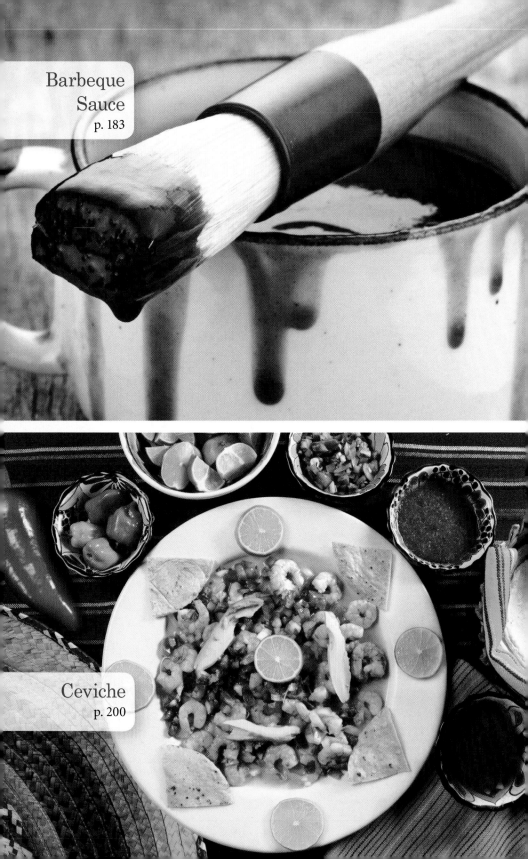

Barbeque
Sauce
p. 183

Ceviche
p. 200

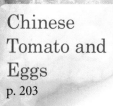

Chicken
Liver Pate'
p. 193

Chinese
Tomato and
Eggs
p. 203

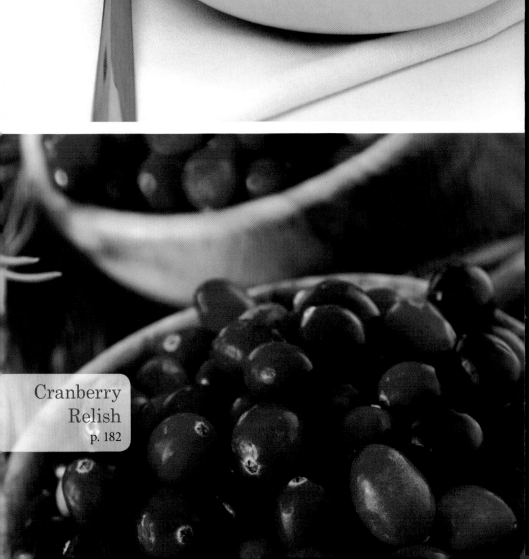

Clam
Chowder
with Bacon
and Green
Chiles
p. 197

Cranberry
Relish
p. 182

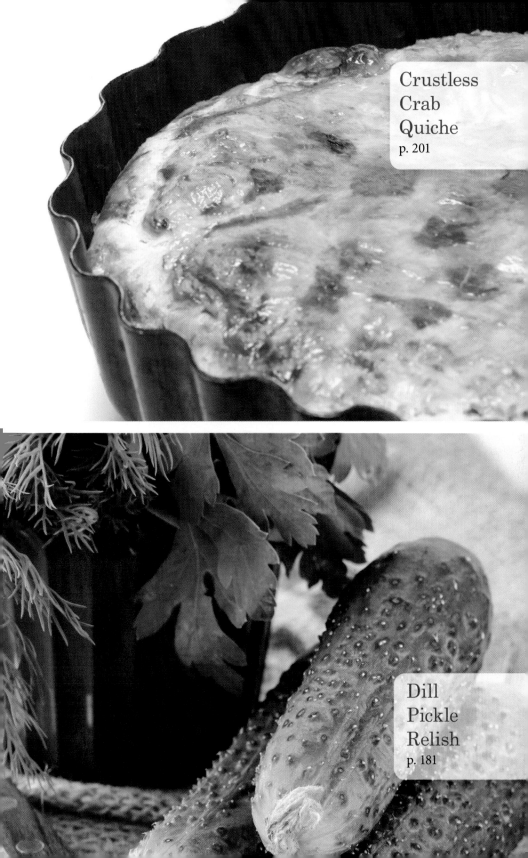

Crustless
Crab
Quiche
p. 201

Dill
Pickle
Relish
p. 181

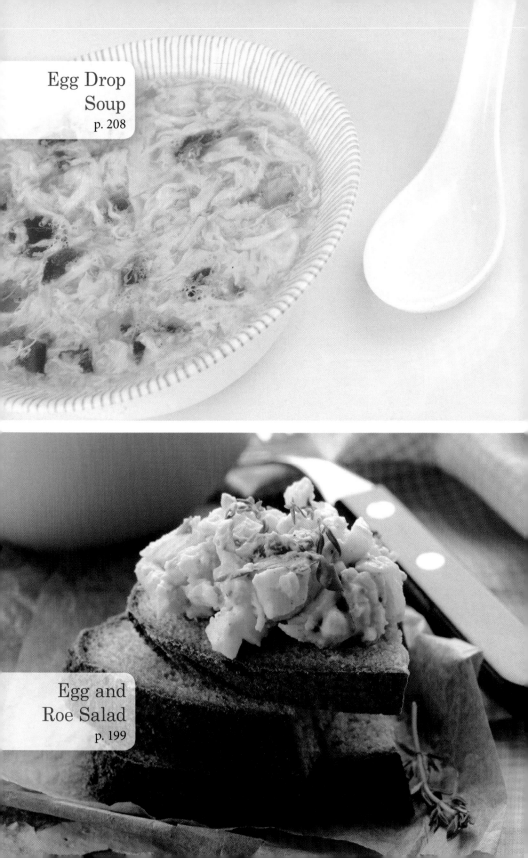

Egg Drop
Soup
p. 208

Egg and
Roe Salad
p. 199

Eggs
Poached in
Marinara
p. 207

Egg-Stravagant
Breakfast
Smoothie
p. 208

Feta Egg
Scramble
p. 210

Fizzy
Lemonade
p. 211

Blender
Hollandaise
Sauce
p. 183

Homemade
Almond
Milk
p. 212

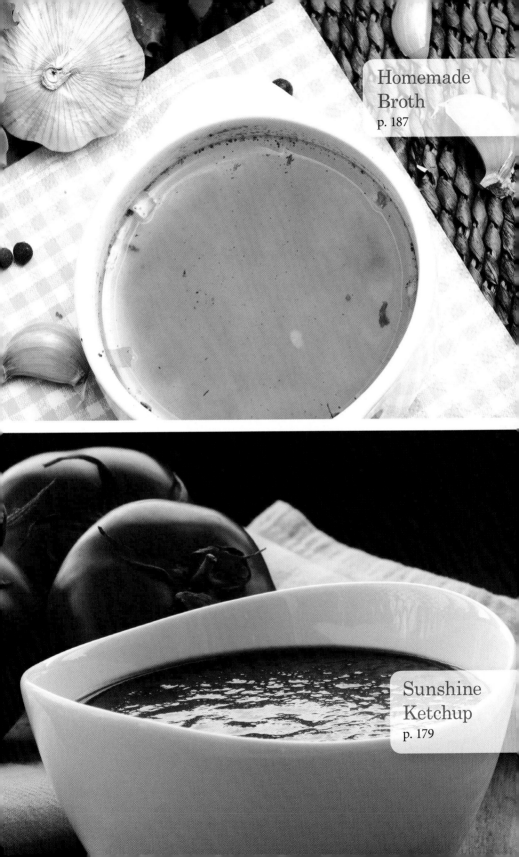

Homemade
Broth
p. 187

Sunshine
Ketchup
p. 179

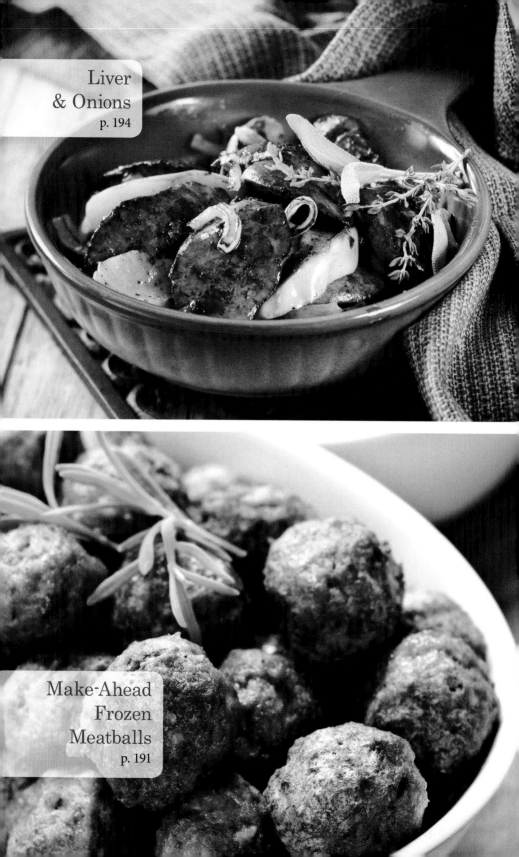

Liver
& Onions
p. 194

Make-Ahead
Frozen
Meatballs
p. 191

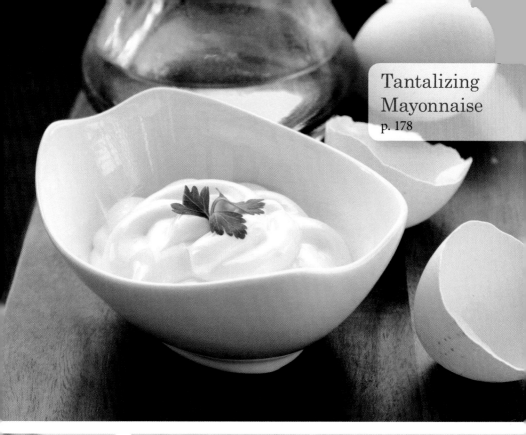

Tantalizing
Mayonnaise
p. 178

Parmesan
Crisps
p. 186

Smoked
Salmon
Mousse
p. 202

Scallops
and Bacon
p. 199

Beef Tongue
Taco Meat
p. 196

Homemade
Taco
Seasoning
p. 185

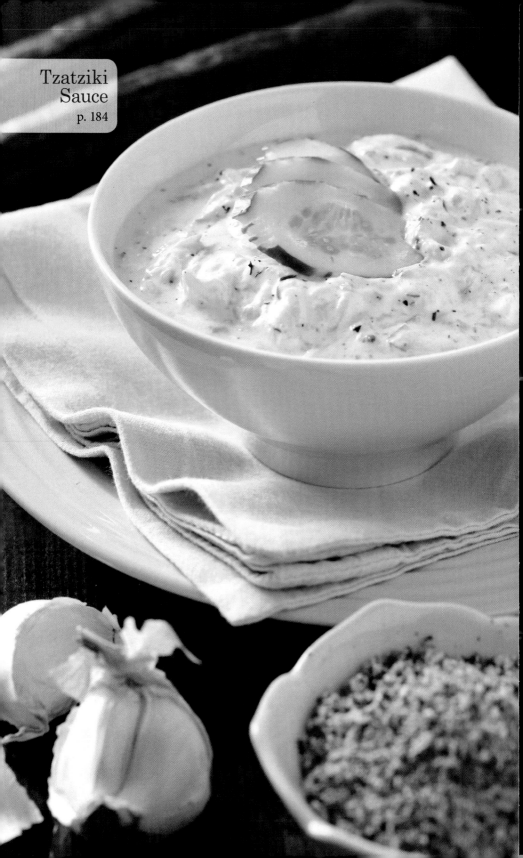

Tzatziki
Sauce
p. 184

Chapter 11

Snacks and Condiments

Probiotic Whey & Greek Yogurt

Cultured foods often require a jump start—a starter culture—to give them a boost of good bacteria. You can buy a vegetable starter culture online, do a "wild" ferment using the naturally present bacteria and yeast in your surroundings, or use the whey drained from a probiotic dairy ferment like kefir or yogurt.

INGREDIENTS

1 quart yogurt or kefir with live, active cultures

EQUIPMENT

Large bowl or small mixing bowl

Kitchen towel (cheesecloth, handkerchiefs, or clean & thin cloth diapers work, too)

Elastic band

DIRECTIONS

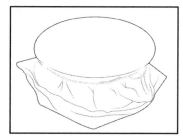

Drape a towel over the bowl, stretch taut, and secure the fabric around the bowl with an elastic rubber band.

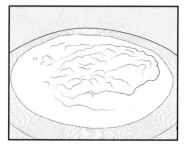

Pour the quart of yogurt or kefir into the towel and let it drip into the bowl.

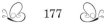

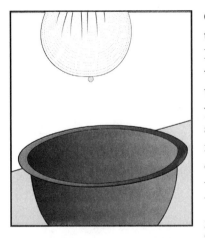

Once the dripping slows, string up the towel to let the whey continue to drip. Leave it until it stops dripping. The time will vary based on the weave of your towel. Untie the towel. What's inside your bowl is probiotic whey, a good starter culture for many fermented foods. You can pour it into a glass jar, cover tightly with a lid, and keep it in your refrigerator for up to a month. What's inside your towel is Greek Yogurt or Labneh. You can use it to make Tzatziki Sauce, Smoked Oyster Spread, Smoked Salmon Mousse, or mix in your own seasonings and herbs for a flavored cheese like dip or spread.

• •

Tantalizing Mayonnaise

INGREDIENTS

2 eggs at room temperature

1 tsp. sucanat/ coconut sugar

1 tsp. raw apple cider vinegar

1 tsp. **Probiotic Whey**

½ cup olive oil

½ cup coconut oil, warmed to liquid

Salt & paprika to taste

EQUIPMENT

Blender

Store-bought mayonnaise is full of industrially processed vegetable oils like soy and canola. Make this homemade mayonnaise with traditional oils instead. You'll not only be getting a tasty mayonnaise free of industrial nastiness, but you'll also be getting a probiotic boost since it's cultured with **Probiotic Whey**.

DIRECTIONS

Put 1 egg and the yolk of the other in your blender, along with sucanat, cider vinegar, & whey. Whirl around for 30 seconds or until nice and frothy. *Slowly* add in olive oil, followed by coconut oil. Add salt and paprika to taste. Transfer to a small, pint sized jar and close the lid tightly. Leave on your counter for 7-12 hours then transfer to the refrigerator and use.

Honey Mustard

Store-bought mustard often contains refined sweeteners. It's also a dead food, made with pasteurized vinegar. This traditionally made mustard packs a probiotic punch and a naturally sour flavor.

DIRECTIONS

Put all ingredients in your food processor and blend until smooth. Transfer to a small, pint sized jar and close the lid tightly. Leave on your counter for two to three days, then transfer to the refrigerator and use.

INGREDIENTS

½ cup whole yellow mustard seeds

⅓ cup water

2 tbsp. raw apple cider vinegar

1 tbsp. honey

2 tbsp. **Probiotic Whey**

1 tsp. salt

1 lemon, juiced

1 clove garlic

EQUIPMENT

Food processor

• •

Sunshine Ketchup

Yet another condiment to fall victim to modern convenience, ketchup used to be cultured with living bacteria to extend its shelf life and create its signature sour taste. Enjoy this full-bodied old-fashioned ketchup instead of a store-bought imitation.

DIRECTIONS

Whisk all ingredients together in a bowl. Transfer to a small glass jar and close the lid tightly. Leave on your counter for two to three days, then transfer to the refrigerator and use.

INGREDIENTS

12 oz. tomato paste

⅓ cup water

2 tbsp. **Probiotic Whey** or vegetable starter culture

2 tbsp. raw apple cider vinegar

2 tbsp. honey

¼ tsp. **Honey Mustard**

⅛ tsp. allspice

½ tsp. salt

Fiesta Salsa

INGREDIENTS

4 tomatoes (medium)

1 jalapeño pepper, seeded

1 onion, peeled and quartered (medium)

1 bunch cilantro

2 cloves garlic

1 lime, juiced

2 tbsp. **Probiotic Whey** or vegetable starter culture

1 tbsp. salt

1 tsp. cumin

1 tsp. oregano

EQUIPMENT

Food processor

Mixing bowl

Homemade salsa with a probiotic kick? Sign me up. This delicious salsa goes well on top of eggs, served alongside fajita salads, or as a dip with (GMO-free!) chips.

DIRECTIONS

Begin by peeling the tomatoes. To do this, boil water on your stove in a large pot. Put your tomatoes in the boiling water for five to ten seconds, then quickly remove with a slotted spoon. When cooled, peel the tomatoes and discard the peel.

Put peppers, cilantro, and garlic in the food processor and pulse until you reach your desired texture. Remove from the food processor and place in a mixing bowl.

Put onion in the food processor and pulse until you reach your desired texture. Remove from the food processor and place in the mixing bowl with the peppers, cilantro, and garlic.

Put tomatoes in the food processor and pulse until you reach your desired texture. Remove from the food processor and place in the mixing bowl with the peppers, cilantro, garlic, and onions.

NOTE: *It is important to pulse ingredients separately in the food processor, otherwise you'll end up with half of your ingredients turning into a puree before the other half is even chopped.*

Add lime juice, whey, salt, cumin, and oregano to the other ingredients in the mixing bowl. Stir until evenly distributed. Transfer to a quart-sized glass jar and seal tightly with a lid. Let rest on your counter for two to three days, then transfer to your refrigerator and eat.

Fresh Tomato Mango Salsa

Sometimes a clever spin on an old favorite charms company or delights your family. I enjoy this tomato mango salsa in the summertime. It's so light, sweet, and divine.

INGREDIENTS

1 cup tomatoes, chopped

½ cup mango, chopped

2 tbsp. cilantro, chopped

1 green onion, diced

1 tbsp. honey

½ lime, juiced

3 tbsp. yogurt, plain

DIRECTIONS

Mix the tomatoes, mango, cilantro, and green onion by hand in a bowl.

In a separate small mixing bowl, combine the honey, limejuice, and yogurt until smooth.

Toss the tomato-mango mixture with the yogurt dressing to create your tomato mango salsa. Refrigerate until ready to serve.

• •

Dill Pickle Relish

When I was a kid, I never liked pickles. That sour vinegar flavor? So off-putting. Thankfully, I discovered old-fashioned "fizzy" pickles—pickles cultured with the wild bacteria in the air to produce a pleasantly sour, crispy delight. Wanting a dill pickle relish free of artificial colors and refined sweeteners, I turned my favorite fizzy pickle recipe into this refreshing condiment.

INGREDIENTS

4-5 pickling cucumbers

2 tbsp. fresh dill (or 2 tsp. dried dill)

2 tbsp. salt

EQUIPMENT

Food processor

DIRECTIONS

Wash cucumbers well & grate them in a food processor or by hand. Stir in remaining ingredients.

Transfer mixture in a quart-sized, wide-mouth mason jar. Using a kitchen mallet or wooden spoon, squeeze the grated cucumbers down and allow liquid to cover them. If there's not enough liquid to cover, add filtered water to get the job done. The top of the liquid should be at least one inch below the top of the jar (that's to make room for all that glorious fermentation).

Cover tightly with a lid and let rest on your counter for 2 days, then transfer to your refrigerator and eat.

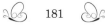

Cranberry Relish

INGREDIENTS

3 cups
cranberries, fresh

1 orange

½ cup pecans,
soaked overnight
in warm, salty
water then dried

½ cup raisins

½ cup orange
juice

½ lemon, juiced

2 tbsp. honey

1 tsp. cinnamon

2 tsp. salt

EQUIPMENT

Food processor

Mixing bowl

Use this rich and flavor-packed, probiotic condiment on sandwiches for a pleasant kick, salads as a dressing, as a dip for things like sliced jicama. Top hamburger patties, cuts of roasted chicken, pork chops, or rice. It's versatile and comforting.

DIRECTIONS

Place cranberries, nuts, and orange in the food processor and pulse until no large chunks remain, but it's not pureed.

Remove from food processor and put in a mixing bowl. Whisk in orange juice, lemon juice, and honey until smooth. Stir in raisins, cinnamon, and salt.

Transfer to a glass, quart-sized jar. Using a wooden spoon or small mallet, press ingredients down until liquid rises to the top. Cover tightly with a lid and let rest undisturbed on your counter for 2 days. Transfer to refrigerator and eat.

• •

Apple Chutney

INGREDIENTS

1 lemon, juiced

1 tbsp. **Probiotic Whey**

½ cup water

3 cups apples, peeled and
chopped coarse

1 tbsp. sucanat or coconut sugar

½ cup walnuts, chopped

½ cup raisins

½ tsp. salt

½ tsp. cinnamon

½ tsp. anise

¼ tsp. cloves

¼ tsp. pepper

I've enjoyed this naturally fermented chutney served on top of oatmeal, alongside steaks and pot roasts, and even just by the spoonful!

DIRECTIONS

Combine all ingredients in a bowl, then transfer to a quart-sized glass jar. Using a wooden spoon or small mallet, press ingredients down until liquid rises to the top. If there's not enough liquid, add more water. Cover tightly with a lid and let rest undisturbed on your counter for a day and a half. Transfer to refrigerator and eat.

Barbeque Sauce

Many store bought barbeque sauces are riddled with corn syrup and industrial cooking oils. Try this homemade version for a healthier alternative.

DIRECTIONS

Melt coconut oil in a saucepan over medium heat. Add onions and cook until tender. Stir in remaining ingredients. Bring to a boil, then reduce heat and simmer for 25 minutes, stirring occasionally. Pour into a glass jar and allow to cool. Cover with a lid and transfer to your refrigerator.

INGREDIENTS

1 tbsp. coconut oil

1 onion, minced (small)

1 tbsp. tamari (naturally fermented soy sauce)

3 cloves garlic, minced

1 tsp. cumin

1 tsp. **Honey Mustard**

1 tsp. basil

1 tsp. oregano

6 oz. tomato paste

1 ¼ cups **Homemade Beef Broth**

2 tbsp. raw apple cider vinegar

2 tbsp. maple syrup

• •

Blender Hollandaise Sauce

The first time I tried this sauce, my taste buds rang out with the Hallelujah chorus. It's a great way to get more nutrient-rich egg yolks from pastured hens in your diet, and it tastes positively sublime. Spoon it over scrambled eggs, poached eggs, steamed veggies. Really, let your imagination run wild.

DIRECTIONS

In your blender's carafe, combine the egg yolks, mustard, and lemon juice. Cover, and blend for about 5 seconds, then remove lid while still blending. Slowly pour the melted butter into the egg yolk mixture in a thin stream, watching it thicken as you slowly pour. Turn off blender. Use sauce immediately.

INGREDIENTS

3 egg yolks

¼ tsp. **Honey Mustard**

3 tsp. lemon juice

½ cup butter, melted

dash cayenne

EQUIPMENT

Blender

Homemade Worcestershire Sauce

INGREDIENTS

½ cup raw apple cider vinegar

2 tbsp. Thai fish sauce

2 tbsp. honey

1 tbsp. molasses

1 lime, juiced

½ tsp. ground clove

½ tsp. onion powder

¼ tsp. garlic powder

¼ tsp. chili powder

Most store bought Worcestershire sauces are heavy on the corn syrup and hidden MSG. This homemade sauce is a fabulous alternative.

DIRECTIONS

Mix all ingredients together in a blender, or shake thoroughly in a dressing bottle! Store in a sealed glass jar in your refrigerator.

• •

Tzatziki Sauce

INGREDIENTS

3 cups **Greek Yogurt**

2 cucumbers, seeded and shredded

1 lemon, juiced

2 cloves garlic, minced

1 tbsp. olive oil

1 tbsp. fresh dill, chopped

Salt, to taste

Refreshing no matter how you serve it, this traditional Greek dip goes great alongside **Make-Ahead Frozen Meatballs**, Greek salads, and lamb. Babies love spooning it into their mouths with sliced carrots and sweet bell peppers.

DIRECTIONS

Begin by lightly salting your seeded and shredded cucumbers. Leave them in a bowl for about 30 minutes to draw out the water. After the half hour has passed, drain the water from your bowl and blot your cucumbers with an absorbent towel.

Whisk all the ingredients together by hand, or use a blender or food processor if you prefer. Transfer to a glass jar, and let refrigerate for at least 2 hours before serving.

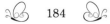 184

Ranch Dressing

A family favorite, typical store-bought ranch dressing boasts a bevy of hidden MSG and industrial oils. Opt for this creamy, tangy dressing instead!

DIRECTIONS

Whisk all ingredients together by hand, or use a blender if you prefer. Transfer to a glass jar, and let refrigerate for at least 2 hours before serving.

INGREDIENTS

1 ½ cups yogurt

4 tsp. olive oil

1 lemon, juiced

2 cloves garlic, minced

1 tbsp. fresh dill, chopped

*½ cup **Tantalizing Mayonnaise***

2 tsp. parsley, chopped

¼ tsp. salt

¼ tsp. onion powder

¼ tsp. pepper

• •

Coconut Almond Dressing

Enjoy this savory dressing as a dip or over salads. Packed full of the good fats you and your growing baby need, it'll satisfy as well as please.

DIRECTIONS

Whisk all ingredients together by hand in a bowl. Serve over salads or as a dip for **Make-Ahead Frozen Meatballs.**

INGREDIENTS

½ cup almond nut butter

½ cup coconut milk

2 tbsp. Thai fish sauce

2 tsp. sesame oil

1 tsp. tamari (naturally fermented soy sauce)

1 tsp. ginger, ground

½ tsp. garlic, ground

• •

Homemade Taco Seasoning

Sadly, store bought taco seasoning is full of nasty stuff with an ingredients label that reads like a chemistry textbook. If you've been wondering how to replace those small packets of MSG-riddled spices with something *real*, you should give this recipe for homemade taco seasoning a try.

DIRECTIONS

Mix all the spices together and store in an airtight container.

INGREDIENTS

1 tbsp. chili powder

¼ tsp. garlic powder

¼ tsp. onion powder

¼ tsp. crushed red pepper flakes

¼ tsp. oregano

½ tsp. paprika

1½ tsp. cumin

1 tsp. sea salt

1 tsp. pepper

Parmesan Crisps

INGREDIENTS

Parmesan cheese, grated (please use REAL Parmesan and not the funky, powdered fake stuff)

If you've ever searched for a healthy alternative to potato chips, you know just how hard they can be to find. It is extraordinarily rare for a store-bought chip to be fried in anything other than an industrially processed, modern, highly-refined vegetable oil. Homemade chips can be made using healthy fats, but they're so much work! As such, they're relegated to ultra-rare treats in our home.

That is, until I discovered Parmesan Crisps! They're so ridiculously easy. Granted, the Parmesan Crisp won't act exactly like your favorite tortilla or potato chip. But as a vehicle for moving delectable dips from a bowl into your mouth, they're pretty yummy and far better than a boring old spoon.

DIRECTIONS

Simply spoon the grated Parmesan cheese into chip-sized, relatively thin dollops on a hot griddle. The cheese will melt, then turn crispy. At this point, use a spatula to flip the crisps over and lightly brown the other side. Then remove from the griddle onto a plate.

The end.

If you don't have a griddle, you can spoon the Parmesan cheese into chip-sized, relatively thin dollops on a cookie sheet or two. Place the cookie sheets in your oven under the broiler and watch them melt and lightly brown. At this point, remove them from the oven and use a spatula to transfer them onto a plate.

The end, again.

When they cool, the Parmesan Crisps will be … crispy. They're perfect for dipping or for using as the base of an appetizer. Enjoy.

Chapter 12
Odd Bits: Organs & Bones

Homemade Broth

DIRECTIONS

Start with the bones. Any bones will do.

Now, some folks will vilify me for this. After all, the kind of bone you use will determine the nutrient-density of the broth as well as the flavor. For the most nutrient-dense and flavorful broth, you want meaty bones with thick marrow (sometimes marketed as "soup bones" by butchers) mixed in with some cut up hooves, knuckles, skull, or feet.

INGREDIENTS

Animal bones— cow bones or a saved chicken or turkey carcass

Water

1 lemon, juiced or 1 tbsp. apple cider vinegar

Salt, to taste

The hooves, knuckles, skull, and feet will help produce the most gelatin-rich broth that's full of other good stuff for your joints (like glucosamine and chondroitin). The meaty bones will produce the hearty flavor you love in a good broth. But the truth is, just about any bones will provide a lot of healthful minerals (like calcium, magnesium, phosphorous, etc.). So, even if you can't get your hands on these super nutrient-dense or flavorful bones, don't fret!

Now, to begin!

First, put the meaty bones in a roasting pan in a 350 degree oven until brown. (You can skip this step if using bones from already roasted meat. Those bones have already experienced the flavor-inducing Maillard reaction necessary for a good broth.) The roasting will create the irresistible flavor and color you expect in a good broth.

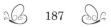

Next put the roasted bones together with the rest of the bones in a stock pot and cover with water. Add a couple of tablespoons of vinegar or lemon juice. The added vinegar or lemon juice will help to draw minerals out of the bones, as well as contribute a subtle flavor that I completely adore in a good broth.

Bring the pot to a boil on the stovetop, then reduce heat to maintain a gentle simmer. Eventually, scum will start rising to the top of the broth. Gently scoop this off and discard it. The rising scum contains many unsavory things, and your broth will be prettier and taste better without it.

Let boil for a long, long time, adding water as needed. The larger the animal, the longer you'll want to cook the broth to get the most nutrients out of the bones. With an animal as large as a cow, that means a full day! With an animal as small as a chicken, you can probably get away with 6-8 hours. Fish only need a couple of hours.

If you want to, add vegetables and salt a few hours before you finish. I never cut up fresh vegetables to add to broth. If I have scraps on hand, or vegetables that need a quick end because they're "starting to turn," then I use them. If not, I don't fret. I always add salt to my broths. That's just a preference of mine. You may choose to do otherwise.

When finished, let the broth cool to room temperature, pick out the large bones, then strain the broth through a wire mesh strainer. Optionally, after the broth is strained you can "condense" it by pouring the strained broth back into your pot and bringing it to a boil to let it reduce further. If using the broth right away (as in a soup), I don't condense it. If making it to use in later culinary delights, then I do. Again, it's just a preference. You do what works for you!

Let the broth cool further in a refrigerator or otherwise cold place. After it's cooled completely, skim the fat off the top and save it for later. That fat is a tasty beef tallow or poultry schmaltz, and you can use it in cooking later. If you don't want to do this step and *want* an oily broth, then skip it. It won't hurt anything, but it may make using the broth in some recipes difficult later.

I store condensed broth two ways: first in quart sized freezer storage bags that can lay flat in my freezer. And second, in ice cube trays! The ice cubes of condensed broth are handy for when I just need a smidgen of flavor added to something (steamed rice, veggies, etc.).

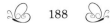

Delectable Roasted Marrow

Loaded with nourishing fats, proteins, and minerals, bone marrow spells heaven on a slice of artisan made sourdough. Babies *and* adults love its meaty flavor and smooth texture. Try it! You'll see.

> **INGREDIENTS**
>
> *Marrow bones*

DIRECTIONS

Preheat oven to 450°F.

Stand your bones up in a roasting tray so that the marrow is exposed and the bone surrounds it. Place in your oven and let roast for 20 minutes, until the marrow is soft and the bones are brown. Remove from oven and let cool slightly.

While still warm, scoop out the marrow with a spoon and serve. Babies almost always *love* roasted marrow. If they had words, they'd be raving about it. To serve to babies, just dish up a few scoopfuls into a small bowl and offer your little one a spoon to go with it. To serve to everyone else, spread on a slice of crusty, real artisan sourdough (not made with commercial yeast or dough conditioners). Enjoy!

Pizza Chili

INGREDIENTS

1 bell pepper, diced

1 onion (small), diced

1 clove of garlic, minced

1 lb. ground beef

½ lb. ground heart*

½ lb. ground liver*

1 small jar sliced black olives

1 package pepperoni (uncured, from humanely raised hogs), sliced & diced

1 quart marinara sauce (homemade, or your favorite organic blend)

*1 quart **Homemade Broth** (chicken)*

Sea salt, basil, red pepper flakes (to taste)

Mozzarella cheese, grated (to taste)

Perhaps the biggest complaint I hear about organ meats like liver is that people just don't like the taste. One of my tricks for getting into my diet is to grind it into ground beef dishes so that it makes up no more than 25% of the total meat. When hidden within a flavorful tomato sauce like the one in this recipe, you can't even taste it.

DIRECTIONS

In a large pot, cook bell peppers, garlic, and onions in a small amount of the fat of your choice until they begin to sweat. Add ground meats and cook until browned.

Stir in olives, optional pepperoni, marinara sauce, and broth. Bring to a boil. Add salt, basil, and red pepper flakes to taste. Allow flavors to mingle over medium heat for 5-10 minutes.

Reduce heat and serve in bowls, topped with mozzarella cheese.

*If you don't have ground versions of these meats, a handy cheat is to grate the frozen (but semi-thawed) meat with a cheese grater.

Make-Ahead Frozen Meatballs

If you've got these meatballs in your freezer, you'll never have an excuse to eat fast food again. The hidden organ meats make them extra nutrient-dense, and you can pop out a few at a time for a quick lunch or dinner. Eat them drenched in marinara or dipped in **Coconut Almond Dressing**. Toss them in a soup. Eat them plain!

INGREDIENTS

3 eggs

1 onion (small), chopped

1 ⅓ cup breadcrumbs (from a real sourdough or sprouted grain bread)

2 ¼ tsp. salt

1 ½ tsp. **Homemade Worcestershire Sauce**

1 tbsp. Italian herb blend

¼ tsp. pepper

2 lbs. ground beef

½ lb. ground liver*

½ lb. ground heart*

DIRECTIONS

Preheat oven to 400°F. In a large bowl, beat the eggs. Add the onions, breadcrumbs, salt, Worcestershire sauce, herbs, and pepper and mix well.

Finally, add the beef, liver, and heart and mix well. Shape the meatballs into one inch balls (should make approximate 100 meatballs).

Place meatballs in single layers on ungreased 1-inch deep baking pans and bake at 400°F for 10 minutes, until done.

Drain the fats and store for later use. (It's grass-fed beef tallow, and it's a wonderful fat to use when cooking.)

Once the meatballs and pans have cooled to the touch, place the meatballs (tray and all) into your freezer to "flash freeze" them. After they've frozen, remove the meatballs from the trays and transfer to plastic freezer storage bags or other freezer storage.

Keep stored in freezer and remove only as many meatballs as you need at a time. You can thank the flash freezing for that. It helps each meatball hold its individual shape and not stick to the other meatballs around it. This way, you can remove as few or as many meatballs as you need for whatever you're serving up.

Reheat the frozen meatballs on the stove, in sauces, or in the oven (350°F for 20 minutes).

*If you don't have ground versions of these meats, a handy cheat is to grate the frozen (but semi-thawed) meat with a cheese grater.

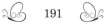

Make-Ahead Frozen Breakfast Sausage Patties

INGREDIENTS

2 tbsp. sage

3 tsp. salt

2 tsp. pepper

1 tsp. marjoram

¼ tsp. crushed red pepper flakes

2 pinches cloves, ground

1 tbsp. molasses

3 lbs. ground pork or beef

1 lb. ground heart*

Store bought breakfast sausages are almost always full of hidden MSG. Instead, you can make these freeze ahead breakfast patties in bulk, then whip them out one at a time as you need to use them. It makes a nourishing, wholesome breakfast just that much quicker to come by. I've used these homemade breakfast sausage patties served alongside eggs, as the base for a down-home Southern gravy, and inside sourdough English muffins to make breakfast sandwiches.

DIRECTIONS

In a bowl, mix all the dry spices.

Next, place the ground meat in a large bowl. Add molasses and dry ingredients. Mix with hands until spices are evenly distributed. Then make patties. (I get about 36 patties out of the 4 pounds of meat.)

Line a cookie sheet with foil or wax paper. Line up your individual patties on the paper so that they're not touching. When the bottom layer is full, add an additional layer of wax paper or foil and keep adding patties. When all the patties are lying flat on the cookie sheet, put the cookie sheet in your freezer. When patties are fully frozen, remove from the cookie sheet and place in a large freezer bag to store for later use.

To cook, sauté the frozen patties over medium heat for approximately 5 minutes per side. Enjoy!

*If you don't have ground heart, a handy cheat is to grate the frozen (but semi-thawed) meat with a cheese grater.

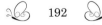

Chicken Liver Paté

Chicken liver has a much more mild taste than beef, and many enjoy cooking them into a paté like this one. If you have a hard time eating beef liver because of its flavor, give this paté a try.

DIRECTIONS

Combine the liver, shallot, garlic, salt and broth in a saucepan. Bring to a simmer.

Cover the pan, reduce the heat to low, and simmer for a few more minutes, stirring once to avoid sticking. Turn off the heat and let stand, covered, for 5 minutes.

INGREDIENTS

½ lb. chicken livers

1 shallot, minced

1 clove of garlic, minced

½ tsp. salt

½ cup **Homemade Broth** (chicken)

⅛ tsp. nutmeg, ground

½ cup butter, softened

EQUIPMENT

Food processor

Transfer to a food processor. Add nutmeg. Pulse until the livers are finely chopped, then add butter a tablespoon or so at a time while you continue to pulse the puree. Blend until completely smooth. Remove from food processor and serve, or let cool in the refrigerator if you prefer cold paté.

Liver & Onions

INGREDIENTS

1 lb. beef liver, sliced

¾ cups milk

¼ cup butter, divided

1 onion (large and sweet), sliced into rings

1 apple, sliced thin

1 cup sprouted-grain flour

Salt and pepper to taste

If you don't mind the flavor of liver, you can't get more down-home and simple than an old-fashioned liver and onions dish. The trick to making these taste fantastic is to soak your liver in milk for a few hours before cooking. This helps "bleed" the liver, making the flavor much milder.

DIRECTIONS

Rinse liver slices with water, then place in a bowl and cover with milk. Let sit for at least two hours, if not more.

In a large skillet, melt 2 tablespoons of butter over medium heat. Sauté onion rings and apples in butter until tender. Remove onions and set aside.

Season the sprouted grain flour with salt and pepper, then pat down onto the surface of a plate.

Melt the remaining butter in the skillet over medium heat. Remove liver slices from milk and coat them in the flour mix.

Turn the heat on your stove up to medium-high. Place the floured liver slices in the buttered pan. Cook until they brown on the bottom, then turn and cook the other side until browned.

Remove immediately from heat and serve with apples and onions on top.

Homemade Braunschweiger

A traditional German paté made with bacon and beef liver. Use in sandwiches, or serve plain.

DIRECTIONS

Rinse liver slices with water, then place in a bowl and cover with milk. Let sit for at least two hours, if not more.

Cook bacon in a large skillet over medium heat. When done, but not crispy, remove and set aside. Save bacon grease in skillet.

Add onions to skillet and cook in grease until tender. Remove onions and set aside.

Add liver slices to skillet and cook in the remaining bacon grease. Cook until they brown on the bottom, then turn them and cook the other side. Remove from heat and place in mixing bowl. Sprinkle with dried, ground spices and stir.

INGREDIENTS

1 lb. beef liver, sliced

¾ cups milk

1 lb. bacon (uncured)

1 onion (small), minced

½ cup cream, divided

1 tbsp. salt

1 tsp. cloves

1 tsp. coriander

1 tsp. nutmeg

½ tsp. sage

¼ tsp. allspice

¼ tsp. cardamom

¼ tsp. pepper

EQUIPMENT

Food processor

Divide bacon, onions, and liver in half. Add first half to food processor and pulse with half the cream until smooth. Empty food processor and blend the second half. Combine both halves in a glass storage container and let cool in refrigerator before serving.

Fried Sweetbreads

INGREDIENTS

1 lb. beef sweetbreads

½ cup sprouted grain flour

1 cup coconut oil or beef tallow

Salt and pepper to taste

Sweetbreads are the perfect organ meat to try for people new to eating odd bits. They've got an appealing, soft texture and taste mildly sweet all on their own.

DIRECTIONS

Sweetbreads will come bunched together with stringy ligaments. In a clean kitchen sink, under running cool water, pull the sweetbread apart into 1 inch sections and discard the ligaments.

In a large skillet, begin melting oil or tallow over medium heat.

Pat the sprouted flour onto the surface of a plate. Cover the slightly wet sweetbreads in the flour.

Fry the floured sweetbreads in the melted oil until they turn golden brown, turning at least once. Remove from oil, and drain on paper towels. Season with salt and pepper to taste.

• •

Beef Tongue Taco Meat

INGREDIENTS

1 beef tongue

1 quart **Homemade Broth** (beef)

½ onion, sliced

5 cloves garlic, crushed

1 tbsp. chili powder

¼ tsp. crushed red pepper flakes

¼ tsp. oregano

½ tsp. paprika

1½ tsp. cumin

1 tsp. salt

EQUIPMENT

Slow-cooker

Tacos de Lengua are a traditional Mexican taco. The meat is easy to prepare in a slow cooker, and it makes a fantastic shredded beef taco meat for use in tacos, burritos, or taco salads.

DIRECTIONS

Put all ingredients together in a slow-cooker set on low. Let cook at least 8 hours. Peel off the outer layer of skin on the tongue. Shred the meat and serve.

Chapter 13

Seafood

Clam Chowder with Bacon and Green Chiles

My husband calls this "New England Clam Chowder Meets Texas." It's a typical clam chowder, but with an extra savory kick. I add bacon to my aromatic vegetables and diced green chilies to my broth base. Oh. My. Goodness.

DIRECTIONS

Begin by frying the bacon in a medium cast-iron skillet. Rather than crumbling hot bacon after it's cooked, I prefer to just cut my raw bacon with kitchen shears and allow it to fry into already-crumbled bits. To your fried bacon bits, add the onion and celery and allow to cook until the veggies turn translucent.

Meanwhile, bring chicken broth to boil in a 6 quart soup pot and add diced potatoes, green chili peppers, taco seasoning, cumin, and salt. Allow potatoes to cook in the boiling broth.

INGREDIENTS

8 slices bacon (uncured)

1 onion (medium), minced

3 stalks celery, chopped

4 potatoes (medium), diced into bite sized pieces

2 quarts **Homemade Broth** (chicken)

8 oz. diced green chili peppers

1 tbsp. **Homemade Taco Seasoning**

1 tbsp. cumin

Salt, to taste

¾ cups butter

¾ cups of sprouted flour

1 quart cream

2 (6.5 oz.) jars clams, minced

8 oz. sour cream

6 oz. cheddar cheese, grated

1 bunch cilantro, chopped (optional)

About 10 minutes before broth and aromatic veggies are ready, begin making your roux in a small saucepan. Melt butter over medium heat; then add flour, stirring constantly to create a pasty roux. To the hot roux, add cold cream. (REMEMBER: HOT roux + COLD cream = NO LUMPS!) Continue stirring over medium heat until it thickens into a nice, creamy gravy.

Transfer bacon and aromatic veggies into your large soup pot. Add thickened gravy to the large soup pot. Stir until evenly mixed. Remove from heat. Add clams and sour cream and stir until evenly mixed.

Serve up your extra tasty clam chowder in bowls, topped with grated cheese and cilantro!

● ●

Crab Salad with Cranberries

INGREDIENTS

6 oz. crabmeat (in glass jars, or a BPA-free can)

2-3 tbsp. **Tantalizing Mayonnaise**

2 tbsp. **Dill Pickle Relish**

1 tbsp. sunflower seeds, soaked overnight in warm, salty water, then dried

2 tbsp. dried cranberries

Refreshingly light and cool, this salad whips together quickly to be a protein-filled treat on days when you don't want to cook.

DIRECTIONS

Mix all ingredients together and serve!

Scallops and Bacon

A surprisingly pleasant combination of flavors accents the nutty undertone of bay scallops—a perfect introduction to this nutrient-rich seafood for those who've never tried them.

DIRECTIONS

Cut bacon with kitchen shears into bite-sized bits. Cook in an iron skillet on medium-high until crisp but not dry. Transfer the bacon to a paper towel or dish.

In a small bowl, combine 1 tbsp. melted coconut oil and 1 tbsp. of limejuice. Coat scallops in the oil mixture, adding salt and pepper to taste.

Transfer scallops to warmed skillet and continue cooking for until opaque, usually about 3 minutes or so. Remove scallops and set aside.

Add the rest of the limejuice to the warmed skillet and begin to scrape the brown bits from the bottom of the pan. Add rosemary, then reserved bacon and scallops. Stir everything around in skillet to coat. Cook about one minute longer to allow flavors to combine, then serve.

INGREDIENTS

2 slices bacon (uncured)

½ lb. bay scallops

1-2 tbsp. coconut oil, divided

Salt & pepper to taste

1 lime, juiced & divided

1 tbsp. rosemary, fresh

• •

Egg and Roe Salad

If you're scared of eating fish roe, don't be. Try out this simple egg salad, laced with whitefish roe—a perfect food for adults and babies alike.

DIRECTIONS

Combine all ingredients in a bowl. Using a fork and knife, smash the eggs while blending all ingredients. When slightly chunky, serve.

INGREDIENTS

6 eggs, hard-boiled

*2 tbsp. **Tantalizing Mayonnaise***

*2 tbsp. **Dill Pickle Relish***

1 oz. whitefish roe

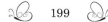

Smoked Oyster Spread

INGREDIENTS

2 4 oz. cans smoked oysters, drained (find BPA-free cans, if possible)

1 ½ cups **Greek Yogurt**

1 tsp. **Homemade Worcestershire Sauce**

Salt & pepper, to taste

If you've ever stared at a fresh oyster still in the shell debating whether or not it's worth the trouble to open them up, you'll be glad to know that there are companies out there canning smoked oysters in BPA-free cans, including Crown Prince Natural and Vital Choice. All you've got to do is whip open a can, and you've got the base for this thick, smoky cheese like spread. Serve on **Parmesan Crisps**, crackers, or sliced veggies.

DIRECTIONS

In a bowl, mash the smoked oysters with a fork. Mix in yogurt, Worcestershire sauce, and salt & pepper. Serve chilled.

• •

Ceviche

INGREDIENTS

8 oz. oysters, chopped

8 oz. salad shrimp

8 limes, juiced

2 tomatoes (large), diced

5 green onions, minced

½ bell pepper, diced

1 bunch parsley, chopped

1 bunch cilantro, chopped

1½ tbsp. olive oil

Pepper, to taste

Cool, refreshing, and ambrosial. That's what ceviche is to me. It's a traditional Latin-American dish made with raw seafood that's "cooked" by the juice of fresh limes. It's light, yet filling, and oh so nutrient-dense.

DIRECTIONS

Rinse raw oysters and shrimp and place in glass bowl and cover with limejuice. Let chill for at least a few hours, or overnight, until oysters and shrimp are opaque.

Pour out half of the limejuice from the bowl. Add diced tomatoes, green onions, bell peppers, parsley, cilantro, olive oil, and pepper to the shrimp and oysters. Stir gently until everything's mixed. Serve cold in glass containers (margarita glasses are fun) for presentation.

Sautéed Oysters With Fennel Butter

Butter and fennel compliment oysters in this surprisingly quick dish. Enjoy it as a main dish, served alongside roasted beets or savory green beans.

INGREDIENTS

1 tsp. ground fennel

1 cup butter, softened

1 shallot (small), minced

½ tsp. cayenne pepper

½ tsp. salt

24 oysters, fresh & shelled

DIRECTIONS

Heat the butter in a medium skillet over medium heat. When melted, add the fennel and shallot. Cook until the shallot is tender. Increase the heat to medium-high and add the oysters. Toss and coat with the butter, then cook until the oysters curl. Remove from heat and sprinkle with cayenne and salt. Serve warm.

• •

Crustless Crab Quiche

Why bother with crusts when you can enjoy a decadent quiche like this?

INGREDIENTS

4 eggs

1 cup cream

½ tsp. salt

½ tsp. pepper

1 cup Monterrey Jack cheese, grated

¼ cup Parmesan cheese, grated

12-16 oz. crabmeat, flaked

1 green onion, chopped

DIRECTIONS

Preheat oven to 350ºF. In a large bowl, whisk together the eggs, cream, salt, and pepper. Stir in grated cheeses, crabmeat, and green onion.

Grease a nine-inch pie dish with either coconut oil or olive oil. Pour quiche mixture into pie dish.

Bake in the oven for 30 minutes. Turn off the oven, but leave the door closed. Leave quiche in the closed oven for an additional 20 to 25 minutes until firm. Remove from oven and serve warm.

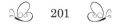

Grilled Crab & Broccoli Cheese Sandwiches

INGREDIENTS

For each sandwich, you'll need:

2 slices sourdough or sprouted grain bread

1 tbsp. smoked Gouda, grated

1 oz. crabmeat, flaked

1 tbsp. steamed broccoli, shredded or finely chopped

1 tbsp. **Tantalizing Mayonnaise**

Butter

You will be utterly shocked that you didn't think of this recipe before. Combine broccoli and cheese with flaked crab and you get a spectacular new take on an ooey, gooey comfort food.

DIRECTIONS

If cooking more than one sandwich, preheat a griddle to medium-high heat. If cooking for just yourself, heat a cast iron skillet over medium.

Assemble the filling. Mix the shredded smoked Gouda, crabmeat, broccoli, and mayonnaise together in a small bowl. Spread between two slices of sourdough or sprouted grain bread and make a sandwich.

Heavily butter both sides of the sandwich. Grill for 3-4 minutes per side. Remove from heat and enjoy!

• •

Smoked Salmon Mousse

INGREDIENTS

4 oz. smoked salmon

2 tbsp. cream

8 oz. **Greek Yogurt**

½ lemon, juiced

½ tsp. dill

Salt and pepper to taste

1 oz. salmon roe

EQUIPMENT

Food processor or blender

Smoked salmon may just be the quintessential deli seafood. Blended in this rich and probiotic mousse, it becomes a culinary masterpiece. Babies and adults enjoy this by the spoonful or with **Parmesan Crisps.**

DIRECTIONS

Blend smoked salmon in a blender or food processor until smooth. Mix in heavy cream, Greek yogurt, lemon juice, dill, salt, and pepper. Pulse a few more times until smooth and thoroughly mixed. Transfer to a serving bowl and garnish with salmon roe.

Chapter 14

Eggs

Chinese Tomato and Eggs

Chinese Tomato and Eggs have long been one of my favorite, simple, hearty dishes. I grew up in the China Town of Houston, in and out of my friends' kitchens, watching hunched over Chinese mothers and grandmothers make everything from simple stir-fries to egg rolls to steamed biscuits. Chinese Tomato and Eggs have always struck me as humble, almost peasant fare. But boy are they tasty!

INGREDIENTS

6 eggs

¼ tsp. toasted sesame oil

salt and white pepper, to taste

2 tomatoes (small), quartered

Water

1 green onion, chopped

Butter

DIRECTIONS

Heat butter in a skillet or wok over medium heat. Mix eggs, sesame oil, salt & pepper in a bowl, then pour into hot skillet. Spread the eggs well with a spatula. Cook as you would scrambled eggs, then remove the eggs and place into a bowl.

Add more butter to the wok or skillet. When melted, stir in tomatoes and green onion. If the tomatoes are juicy, just cover them and cook for about 30 seconds. If they're not a particularly juicy variety, sprinkle a tablespoon or so of water on the tomatoes before covering and cooking for about 30 seconds. Remove the cover, add the scrambled eggs, and cook for an additional 30 seconds or a minute until the tomatoes are hot and tender but not overly cooked. Serve immediately.

Grain-Free Apple Pancake Rings

INGREDIENTS

3 eggs

3 tbsp. coconut oil

3 tbsp. milk or coconut milk

1 tsp. honey

½ tsp. salt

1 tsp. cinnamon

3 tbsp. coconut flour

2 apples (medium), sliced thin and cored

Because these "pancakes" are made with coconut flour, they need an abundance of eggs to have the right cake-like texture. Putting eggs into foods like this is a delicious way to enjoy eggs. Not all egg dishes have to be savory.

DIRECTIONS

In a mixing bowl, whisk together eggs, coconut oil, milk, honey, cinnamon, and salt. Once evenly mixed, whisk in coconut flour. Stir until evenly mixed, then let sit for 5 minutes.

Heat a griddle or cast iron skillet to medium heat. Melt a dab of coconut oil on your cooking surface. While that's heating and your batter is resting (an essential step when working with coconut flour), this is a good time to peel, slice, and core your apples if you haven't already.

Using a toothpick, pick up an apple ring and dunk it in the pancake batter. Then, put it on the griddle. Repeat for as many apple pancake rings as you've got room to cook. Once the batter has cooked firm around the edges and turned golden brown, flip once to cook the other side to golden brown.

When finished, serve apple pancake rings warm. We love serving it up with slices of cheese, or with a natural syrup like sorghum or maple.

Basil Eggs Ringed in Bell Pepper

Eggs from pastured hens are fried with basil in coconut oil, INSIDE a slender, tender ring of bell pepper. Top it with a dollop of sour cream and a pinch of salt, and you have an easy fried egg with lots of eye-appeal!

INGREDIENTS

Eggs, one for each bell pepper ring

1 yellow bell pepper, cut into 1/3 inch wide rings

Coconut oil

Basil, fresh, one leaf for each ring

Sour cream, one dollop for each ring

Salt, to taste

DIRECTIONS

Begin by warming your cast iron skillet up to medium low while melting your coconut oil. After the fat melts, put your bell pepper rings flat in the pan. Allow to cook for a few minutes, then flip.

Place a basil leaf inside each cooking bell pepper ring. Crack eggs open into your rings. Some whites may leak from under the bottom of your rings. Not to worry. Just press down on your rings with a spatula to minimize spread and help the edges "set."

Allow eggs to cook until desired wellness. I usually wait until the egg whites have set, then cover my cast iron skillet with a lid or a plate to trap the heat in and allow the egg yolk to firm up. (This makes it so I don't have to flip an egg to get a yolk cooked medium or hard.)

Remove eggs from skillet. Top with sour cream and a sprinkling of salt.

Texas Style Crustless Quiche

INGREDIENTS

6 slices bacon
(uncured)

1 sweet onion
(medium), diced

1 red bell pepper, diced

10 oz. baby spinach

8 oz. of grated cheddar

5 eggs

½ cup milk

Ground chipotle
pepper to taste

Coconut oil

In this crustless quiche recipe, the savory flavor of bacon blends seamlessly with the spicy heat of chipotle pepper. The accents of Texas Vidalia sweet onions and sweet red bell peppers round out the dish and give it that famous Texas "kick."

DIRECTIONS

In a cast iron skillet, grill bacon over medium heat until cooked. Remove bacon from skillet and add onions & red bell peppers. Cook until onion becomes translucent. Add spinach and stir until wilted. Remove pan from heat, stir bacon back into mix.

In the meantime, mix cheese, eggs, milk, and chipotle pepper in a medium mixing bowl. Add vegetable and bacon mix and stir until blended.

Grease a nine-inch pie dish with your fat of choice. (I use coconut oil.) Pour quiche mixture into pie dish. Bake at 375ºF for 40-45 minutes or until filling is set. Let rest for 10 minutes before serving.

Eggs Poached in Marinara

Who needs pasta, anyway? Eggs poached in marinara sauce are the way to go! They may not look "pretty," but they take mere minutes to prepare. And they're delicious.

INGREDIENTS

Eggs, as many as you want to serve

1 cup of marinara sauce per egg.

DIRECTIONS

In a deep dish skillet bring marinara sauce to a boil over medium heat. Reduce the heat to medium low so that the sauce is no longer bubbling.

With a spoon, create "slots" for your eggs—tiny indentations in the marinara that will act like "bowls" in the sauce and hold your eggs in their places. Crack open one egg per slot.

Now for the truly difficult part: Cover the skillet with your lid and be patient. Cook eggs until they reach your desired consistency. I personally love them with runny yolks, but my kiddos love them cooked hard.

Spoon eggs and a generous portion of sauce into serving bowls. Enjoy!

Egg Drop Soup

INGREDIENTS

1 onion, diced

2 stalks celery, diced

1 tbsp. butter

8 cups **Homemade Broth** (chicken)

¼ tsp. ground ginger

1 tsp. tamari (naturally fermented soy sauce)

¼ tsp. sesame oil

Salt to taste

3 tbsp. arrowroot powder (or corn starch) + 3 tbsp. water

6 eggs

It's fast. It's nutritious. It's Egg Drop Soup.

DIRECTIONS

Dice onions and celery. Melt butter over medium heat. Sauté onions & celery over low heat until they turn soft.

Stir in broth. Add ginger, tamari, and sesame oil. Bring to a boil. Add salt to taste.

Mix arrowroot powder or cornstarch with water until smooth. Pour into soup and cook until thickened.

Whisk your eggs together and pour intermittently into soup. For beautiful, ribbony eggs be sure to do this step after the soup is already thickened!

• •

Egg-Stravagant Breakfast Smoothie

INGREDIENTS

2 eggs, plus 2 egg yolks

1 banana

1 cup berries (frozen) of choice

1 cup yogurt

1 tsp. honey

Milk

Smoothies are one of my favorite ways to eat eggs when I don't want a savory breakfast. They're cool, sweet, but loaded with all the vitamins, fats, and proteins you need to get a great start to your morning.

DIRECTIONS

Put all ingredients in your blender. Add enough milk to cover. Blend until smooth. Add milk to thin the smoothie, if desired, then pulse a few additional times to mix well. Pour into drinking glasses and enjoy immediately.

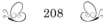

Summer Squash Omelet with Tomato Gravy

DIRECTIONS

In a skillet, sauté yellow squash in 1 tbsp. olive oil over medium heat until it becomes tender.

Put tomatoes in a small saucepan, cover, and cook over medium heat in their own liquid until they soften.

In a bowl, whisk eggs together. Add cooked squash to the eggs and mix. Warm another tbsp. of olive oil in the skillet. Lift skillet and spread it around, helping it to coat the bottom of the pan. Pour egg mixture back into warmed skillet and let cook for one minute. Put a lid on the skillet and cook 1-2 minutes more, or until firm. (Hint: if your skillet doesn't come with a lid, use a dinner plate.)

While your omelet cooks, move tomatoes to the edges of the bottom of the saucepan, clearing a space in the middle. Add butter. When that melts, add sprouted grain flour to the butter and stir until all the flour has absorbed butter. Now, pour in cold milk and continue stirring as the gravy thickens to desired consistency. Add honey, plus salt and pepper to taste.

If you haven't already, remove cooked omelet from the skillet to your plate. Ladle tomato gravy over the omelet and serve immediately.

INGREDIENTS

1 yellow squash, peeled and shredded

4 eggs

2 tomatoes, diced

2 tbsp. olive oil, divided

1 tbsp. butter

1 tbsp. sprouted grain flour

½ cup milk

1 tsp. honey

Salt and pepper, to taste

Feta Egg Scramble

INGREDIENTS

1 tbsp. butter

½ onion (medium), chopped

4 eggs, beaten

1 tomato (medium), diced

2 tbsp. feta cheese, crumbled

Salt and pepper, to taste

Think scrambled eggs couldn't get any more boring? You haven't had them with feta melted into them.

DIRECTIONS

Melt butter in a skillet over medium heat. Add onions, sauté until tender and translucent. Pour in eggs. Continue cooking over medium heat, stirring occasionally to scramble the eggs. When eggs are almost done, stir in tomatoes and crumbled feta cheese. Add salt and pepper to taste. Cook until cheese is melted.

• •

Tomato Parmesan Egg Cupcakes

INGREDIENTS

12 eggs

⅓ cup milk

1 tomato (medium), diced

1 tbsp. olive oil

5 **Make-Ahead Frozen Breakfast Sausage Patties**

½ cup Parmesan, grated

½ tsp. basil, dried

These make a quick grab-n-go breakfast or snack. Make a large batch, then keep in your fridge for later in the week.

DIRECTIONS

Preheat oven to 325°F.

In a large skillet, cook the frozen breakfast sausage patties, browning them and breaking them apart as they cook.

While the sausage is cooking, whisk together the eggs and milk in a large mixing bowl. Add tomatoes, Parmesan, basil, and browned sausage to mixing bowl and stir until well mixed.

Use olive oil to grease cupcake tins. Ladle the egg mixture into cupcake tins. Bake in preheated oven for 25-30 minutes, or until cooked through.

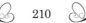

Chapter 15

Beverages

Fizzy Lemonade

It's like lemonade, but with pizazz and a probiotic wallop.

DIRECTIONS

Put all ingredients together in a one gallon glass container and stir well. Cover tightly with a lid and let sit on your counter at room temperature for two days. It is now ready to drink or refrigerate.

INGREDIENTS

12 lemons, juiced

1 cup sucanat or coconut/palm sugar

*1 cup **Probiotic Whey***

1 gallon water

• •

Homemade Orange Soda

Sweet and zingy, fizzy and light. Drink this probiotic tonic instead of store-bought sodas.

DIRECTIONS

Put all ingredients in a half gallon glass jar. Cover tightly with a lid and let sit on your counter at room temperature for two days. It is now ready to drink or refrigerate. Stir well before serving.

INGREDIENTS

12 oranges, juiced

2 tsp. salt

*¼ cup **Probiotic Whey***

½ tsp. orange extract

1¾ quarts water

Homemade Almond Milk

INGREDIENTS

1 ½ cups almonds, soaked in warm, salty water overnight, then drained and rinsed

4 cups water

3-5 dates

EQUIPMENT

Blender

If you can't find grass-fed milk but still want to drink a milk-like beverage, you may opt for a nut milk. If you do, it's best to make it at home. Store bought almond milks usually contain added sugars, preservatives, and stabilizers. Plus, almonds also contain the anti-nutrient phytic acid which can block mineral absorption. You can neutralize the phytic acid by soaking the almonds overnight—something you're not likely to be able to find in store-bought versions.

DIRECTIONS

Put all ingredients into a blender and blend. Strain once with a fine mesh strainer to remove almond granules, and enjoy your drink.

• •

Homemade Flavored Kombucha

INGREDIENTS

1 gallon sweetened tea

1 kombucha mother (AKA "scobies," or "mushrooms")

7 oz. of fruit juice

EQUIPMENT

1 gallon glass jar

1 thin kitchen towel plus a rubber band

3 quart-sized glass jars with lids (any size bottle or jar will do, so long as you've got enough to hold 75%-80% of your brewed kombucha)

Kombucha is a fizzy, mildly sweet and tart health drink that works wonders detoxing our bodies. When you're craving a fizzy energy boost without the sugar crashes that accompany a soda habit, kombucha will satisfy. A sixteen ounce store-bought bottle of organic raw kombucha costs around $3.50. Multiply that times several family members and a couple of glasses per day, and it adds up quickly.

If you could brew your own flavored kombucha for as little as $1.50/gallon and about ten minutes of your time, why wouldn't you?

DIRECTIONS

Some Important Notes Before You Start:

First—Assuming you didn't grow your own mother, you've got a week to ten days to start this process from the day you receive the kombucha starter or "mother" to ensure the freshest and most healthful product. If you let the mother sit too long in your refrigerator it will make the kombucha stale.

Second—Each mother comes with at least a half a cup of liquid with it. That is important stuff so do not pour it off. You'll actually use that in your first batch of tea. I recommend buying a bottle of Kombucha from the health food store to help your first batch, but this isn't necessary. If you choose to do it, you'll want to buy Organic Raw Kombucha without any fruit sweeteners added.

Finally—The starter is a bit strange and takes some getting used to. Handling it and placing it on top of the tea just takes a little practice and a sense of adventure ... it is pretty disarming initially.

One final note—EVERYONE will tell you something different. Brewing kombucha is just like making any other dish. There are hundreds of variations and recipes out there, each one somebody's favorite. Everyone will swear doing this or that particular thing will make the beverage more healthful for you—and often the advice is contradictory. My point? Relax. Just do it. Enjoy it. Experiment and see what works for you.

Day 1 / Part One: Make Sweetened Tea

Boil about 1 gallon of fresh, filtered water on the stovetop. Once water is at a full boil, remove from heat and add tea bags or family-sized tea bag and steep for 5 minutes. You can use plain black tea for this, or experiment with other black or green teas as you desire.

Remove tea bags and add 1 cup of sugar stirring vigorously until it is dissolved. (This is the only thing in my house we use refined sugar for. We tried brewing kombucha with natural sweeteners like sucanat or honey, but they all made the final brew take longer and taste sour. There's no need to fear this refined sugar because it's basically just food for the yeast.) Let the sweetened tea sit on the stovetop until it has cooled to room temperature. This usually takes about 2 hours.

Day 1 / Part Two: Add the Mother to the Sweetened Tea

Once tea is cooled down, transfer to glass jar with a wide mouth. (The kombucha doesn't brew as well in metal or plastic containers. You can use a large glass bowl, glass pitchers, or a large glass sun tea jar—anything glass that will hold your tea.) Pour the half cup of liquid that comes with the mother into the sweetened tea.

Carefully place the mother on top of the tea mixture.

Cover your glass containers with a clean kitchen towel and place away from direct sunlight. I secure the towel with large rubber bands. The kombucha needs oxygen to ferment, so you're using a towel rather than a lid to allow air to circulate. The rubber band secures the towel to keep out flies, insects, or other contaminants.

Days 1-5: Ferment Tea

You will allow the tea mixture to set out in the dark corner of your kitchen for 5 days. On the morning of Day 5, remove the mother and set it aside on a plate, pouring about a half cup of the fermented tea mixture over the mother to keep it moist. Put it in the refrigerator. Every other batch or so, you'll be able to separate the old mother from its "baby" which will have grown on top of the old mother. (It may separate on its own, or you may just pull them apart.) When that happens, the baby will become the mother for your next batch of kombucha tea. The "old" mother can be passed on as a gift or discarded.

Day 5 / Part One: Ferment With Fruit Juice

Pour clear fruit juice (no pulp, it causes much stringy nastiness!) into the smaller glass jars or bottles you're using to bottle your kombucha. I use about 2 to 2 ½ ounces of fruit juice per quart-sized jar. You can use any size bottle or jar, just be sure to adjust the fruit juice accordingly.

Pour kombucha tea on top of the fruit juice, allowing about an ounce of breathing room at the top of the bottle, then close bottle tightly. Be sure to save at least 10% of your brewed kombucha to use with your saved mother in your next batch. To ensure a consistent brew, I save about 25% of mine.

Place bottles back in your "fermenting place" for 48 hours and cover with a kitchen towel so they avoid exposure to direct sunlight.

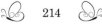

Day 5 / Part Two: Begin Your Next Batch

Repeat the process for Day 1, Parts One and Two, and use the mother you set aside earlier as the mother for this batch of kombucha tea.

Day 7: Finish

Put bottles in the refrigerator and chill completely before opening. Don't shake. When you open, remove the thin film of new "mother" that accumulated on top during the fruit juice fermentation phase. Contents will be bubbly.

Some Final Notes:

Your kombucha mother may turn brown, or bubbly, or do all sorts of strange things. None of these are problems. The only thing you want to really look out for is mold, and if it molds it will look like the mold on bread—fuzz and all.

These instructions are assuming that the room temperature where you're brewing your kombucha is around 75 degrees. (I'm in Texas, what can I say?) *If the temperature is considerably warmer than this, it will take less time to ferment. If it is considerably cooler than this, it will take more time to ferment.* As such, people find that during the winter in cooler climates they may let their kombucha ferment for up to a week longer than they do during the height of summer. How can you tell when your kombucha's ready to be bottled with fruit juice? When it's mildly sweet and mostly tart.

Appendix A:
Understanding Food Ingredient Labels

When buying packaged foods, get in the habit of reading ingredient labels. The main things to look for are:

1. foods containing MSG or free glutamic acids

2. foods containing corn derivatives

3. foods containing GMOs

4. foods containing modern, industrialized oils or fats

5. foods containing artificially created dyes or sweeteners

If a food contains any of these things, then it is a highly processed industrialized food. These are the foods that you want to phase-out of your diet and eliminate completely.

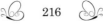

Finding Hidden MSG and Free Glutamic Acids

Ingredients that always contain processed free glutamic acid:

- Glutamic acid (E 620*)
- Glutamate (E 620)
- Monosodium glutamate (E 621)
- Monopotassium glutamate (E 622)
- Calcium glutamate (E 623)
- Monoammonium glutamate (E 624)
- Magnesium glutamate (E 625)
- Natrium glutamate
- Yeast extract
- Anything "hydrolyzed"
- Any "hydrolyzed protein"
- Calcium caseinate
- Sodium caseinate
- Yeast food, Yeast nutrient
- Brewers' yeast
- Autolyzed yeast
- Gelatin (except that made by a specialized process, like Great Lakes brand)
- Textured protein
- Vetsin
- Ajinomoto

Ingredients that often contain free glutamic acids:

- Carrageenan (E 407)
- Bouillon and broth
- Stock
- Whey protein
- Whey protein concentrate
- Whey protein isolate
- Natural flavor
- Any "flavor" or "flavoring"
- Maltodextrin
- Citric acid (E 330)
- Anything "ultra-pasteurized"
- Barley malt, Malted barley
- Pectin (E 440)
- Protease
- Anything "enzyme modified"
- Anything containing "enzymes"
- Malt extract
- Soy milk
- Soy sauce
- Soy sauce extract
- Soy protein
- Soy protein concentrate
- Soy protein isolate
- Anything "protein fortified"
- Anything "fermented"
- Seasonings

These numbers are pharmacy codes for the flavor enhancers and are sometimes used to identify these ingredients on food labels.

Finding Corn Derivatives

- corn syrup
- high-fructose corn syrup
- corn oil
- vegetable oil
- partially hydrogenated corn oil
- ascorbic acid*
- caramel color*
- citric acid*
- corn starch
- crystalline fructose*
- dextrose*
- distilled white vinegar
- ethanol
- fumaric acid*
- lactic acid*
- lecithin*
- maltose*
- modified corn starch
- monosodium glutamate*
- xanthan gum*
- xylitol*

These are not always derived from corn, although they can be.

Finding GMOs

The eight genetically modified food crops in the U.S. are corn, soybeans, canola, cottonseed, sugar beets, Hawaiian papaya (most), and a small amount of zucchini and yellow squash.

Unfortunately, because of our labeling laws (which do not require the labeling of genetically modified foods), the only way to avoid getting genetically engineered versions of these foods is to buy certified organic or from farmers you trust.

Processed food ingredients that can be made from GMOs (unless they are organic or declared non-GMO):

- ascorbic acid (vitamin C)
- Aspartame (also called AminoSweet, NutraSweet, Equal Spoonful, Canderel, BeneVia, E951)
- baking powder
- canola oil (rapeseed oil)
- caramel color
- cellulose
- citric acid
- cobalamin (vitamin B12)
- colorose
- condensed milk
- confectioner's sugar
- corn flour
- corn masa
- corn meal
- corn oil
- corn sugar
- corn syrup
- cornstarch
- cottonseed oil
- cyclodextrin
- cystein
- dextrin
- dextrose
- diacetyl
- diglyceride
- erythritol
- Equal
- food starch
- fructose (any form)
- glucose
- glutamate
- glutamic acid
- glycerides
- glycerin
- glycerol
- glycerol monooleate
- glycine
- hemicellulose
- high-fructose corn syrup (HFCS)
- hydrogenated starch
- hydrolyzed vegetable protein
- inositol
- inverse syrup
- inversol
- invert sugar
- isoflavones
- lactic acid
- lecithin
- leucine
- lysine
- malitol
- malt
- malt syrup

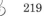

- malt extract
- maltodextrin
- maltose
- mannitol
- methylcellulose
- milk powder
- milo starch
- modified food starch
- modified starch
- mono and diglycerides
- monosodium glutamate (MSG)
- Nutrasweet
- oleic acid
- Phenylalanine
- phytic acid
- protein isolate
- shoyu
- sorbitol
- soy flour
- soy isolates
- soy lecithin
- soy milk
- soy oil
- soy protein
- soy protein isolate
- soy sauce
- starch
- stearic acid
- sugar (unless cane sugar)
- tamari
- tempeh
- teriyaki marinades
- textured vegetable protein
- threonine
- tocopherols (vit E)
- tofu
- trehalose
- triglyceride
- vegetable fat
- vegetable oil
- vitamin B12
- vitamin E
- whey
- whey powder
- xanthan gum

Modern, Industrialized Oils

- Anything "hydrogenated"
- Anything "partially-hydrogenated"
- Corn oil
- Soybean oil
- Soy oil
- Canola oil
- Vegetable oil
- Sunflower oil
- Safflower oil

Artificially Created Dyes & Sweeteners

- Acesulfame potassium (Nutrinova)
- Aspartame (NutraSweet, Equal)
- Salt of aspartame-acesulfame (TwinSweet)
- Glucin
- Neohesperidin dihydrochalcone
- Neotame (NutraSweet)
- Saccharin (Sweet'N Low)
- Sucralose (Splenda, Kaltame)
- Blue No. 1—Brilliant Blue FCF, E133 (blue shade)
- Blue No. 2—Indigotine, E132 (indigo shade)
- Green No. 3—Fast Green FCF, E143 (turquoise shade)
- Red No. 40—Allura Red AC, E129 (red shade)
- Red No. 3—Erythrosine, E127 (pink shade, commonly used in glacé cherries)
- Yellow No. 5—Tartrazine, E102 (yellow shade)
- Yellow No. 6—Sunset Yellow FCF, E110 (orange shade)

Appendix B:
Eating Real Food on a Budget

Even in the best of economic times, my family has always had a rather small budget for food. When my husband and I first got married, we were both full-time students working part-time, minimum wage jobs at $4/hour. There were months when I fed both of us for just $15/week!

Granted, it wasn't particularly real food, but I mostly mention it to say: I've been there, folks. I've been dirt poor trying to do the best I can with what I had.

I understand the sticker shock that comes from choosing nourishing, real foods. It can be hard to pay $8.50 a gallon for grass-fed raw milk when the grocery store milk is $3 a gallon less. It feels *crazy*.

And, it often makes people give up in frustration before they've even begun to incorporate better food choices into their diet. Well, I'm here to tell you it *can be done*. You may not be able to do it all at once; I know we didn't. It's taken us years to get to where we are, and we still make compromises all the time because of budget constraints. So, give yourself a little grace.

There are two components to eating Real Food on a budget. One is learning *what foods to prioritize sourcing well*, and the other is learning *how to manage your kitchen properly* to stretch those dollars.

How to Prioritize Food Choices

Without question, this is how I prioritize spending my money:

1. **Getting High Quality Fats & Oils**—The goal here is to eat a traditional balance of fats by reducing the amount of omega 6 fatty acids in our diet and increasing the amount of omega 3 fatty acids. It's also to eat more saturated and monounsaturated fats, and to reduce polyunsaturated fat intake to less than 4%. You can do that by switching to traditional fats. If buying quality animal fats like lard or tallow from pastured/ wild/grass-fed animals is too expensive, consider using more coconut

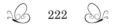

oil, butter, and olive oil in your cooking. Whatever you do, **eliminate all yellow seed oils** like corn oil, vegetable oil, canola oil, etc. If you're worried that you're not getting enough omega 3 oils, despite your best efforts, by all means buy and take a quality fish oil or krill oil supplement that's been certified mercury-free, etc. I *highly recommend* supplementing with fermented cod liver oil, just because of all its wonderful nutritional benefits.

2. **Buying Raw or Fermented Dairy From Grass-Fed Animals**— Obviously, this is a big step, and knowing how to prioritize buying milk or cheese can be difficult. Check out the prioritization I recommend in Chapter 4. Fermented dairy includes yogurt, kefir, cheese, sour cream, buttermilk, and the like. These all contain healthy bacteria and living enzymes.

3. **Getting High Quality Meats, Fish, & Eggs**—By this, I mean for you to eat meats from humanely raised, pastured animals or wild-caught seafood. Grass-fed beef is nutritionally superior to its industrially raised counterpart, and the same can be said for *any* pastured meats. High quality eggs are trickier to find, thanks to lax labeling standards here in the U.S. that allow egg packaging to be quite misleading and downright deceptive. Read Chapter 4 for more on how to prioritize your purchases of meats, fish, and eggs.

4. **Buying Organic Fruits & Veggies**—If you've done the first three things on this list and still have some wiggle room in your budget, then start buying as many organic fruits & veggies as you can afford. Prioritize buying organic on thin-skinned fruits & vegetables like grapes, peaches, leafy greens, etc. If a fruit or vegetable has a thicker-skin or peel, you can feel safer buying non-organic because you can simply peel it and eliminate most pesticides that way.

Please note that buying organic fruits & vegetables is *way down on the list*. In fact, it's got the lowest priority. That's because of all the changes listed above, switching to organic fruits & vegetables will have the smallest effect on your fertility, health and nutritional well-being.

How to Manage Your Kitchen Properly

This is how I manage my kitchen:

1. **I prepare our own meals**—Eating out is a luxury. And contrary to what KFC claimed in their infamous $10 Challenge commercial, it really is cheaper to cook your own food at home.

2. **I don't buy packaged foods**—This is a *huge* money saver! (And it does wonders for your health.) Remember, even so-called "organic" packaged foods can contain unhealthy ingredients like MSG.

3. **I buy in bulk, and directly from local farmers when possible**—I pick up bulk grains and beans and natural sweeteners from my local grocery store (or in buying clubs with like-minded friends & neighbors), and I also plan large once-a-year purchases of pastured beef and poultry. This saves a lot of money. It is considerably cheaper to buy grass-fed meat in bulk than to buy it by the cut, and (with the exception of ground beef) I beat grocery store prices for industrially raised meats for just about every cut of steak or roast out there. I know that having freezer space is an issue for many; it was for me for years. But I kept my eyes peeled for free or low-cost freezers on Craigslist and Freecycle, and eventually ended up getting one when I moved into my new house. Considering that I'm probably saving $850 a year in meat costs alone, even buying a new freezer would pay for itself quickly.

4. **I eat fewer animal products (and more veggies)**—While I believe animal products are far healthier for me than the diet dictocrats would have us believe, I'm also a vegan for about 40% of the year thanks to my religious principles (Orthodox Christian). And, even when I'm not keeping a vegan fast due to pregnancy or breastfeeding, my family of five still only averages about six pounds of meat per week over the course of the year. *The trick here is to make meat only a part of the meal, rather than the centerpiece.* Instead of serving one chicken breast per person with some sides, we'll cut up the chicken and put it in a casserole or soup or on top of a giant salad.

5. **I don't waste food**—We save up unused vegetable parts and uneaten leftovers to make hearty broths and soups each week, use chicken giblets to make gravy, use the carcass for a gelatin-rich broth that's oh-so-good for your joints. This way, I can generally get four meals out of each chicken!

6. **I make my own convenience foods**—Breads, salsas, salad dressings, condiments. It's all healthier and cheaper when you make it at home.

7. **I try not to double up on expensive animal proteins in any given meal**—This means I rarely pair meat with cheese, eggs with cheese, meat with eggs, and the like unless I'm cooking up something special. I save lasagna and quiche for when I have company.

8. **I eat in season & locally, when possible**—This can also save you a significant amount of money. Inevitably, there is always a week at the Farmer's Market when *everyone* has tomatoes. When that happens, they're surprisingly cheap! I'll buy a whole case of them and can them for the winter. The same goes for any other fresh fruit or vegetable. Buy it when it's at the peak of its flavor, and you'll not only pay less, your food will *taste so much better.*

In the past whenever I've shared my exact food budget with others, I've always been amazed by the diversity of people's comments. What I've learned is that food costs vary greatly from place to place. You simply need to do the best you can with what you've got.

With time, you'll start feeling comfortable spending a little more on food and cutting out other expenses that seem less necessary. If you're not there yet, don't worry. Just do your best!

I will conclude with this thought: I feed my family of five nourishing, real food on *far less* than the federal food stamp allotment for a family my size ($793/month). It takes a lot of thought, planning, and detective work to eat this way, but I do it.

Endnotes

Chapter 1: Paradigm Shifts

1. Pollan, Michael. *Food Rules: An Eater's Manual.* Camberwell, Vic.: Penguin, 2010. Print.

2. Planck, Nina. *Real Food for Mother and Baby: The Fertility Diet, Eating for Two, and Baby's First Foods.* New York: Bloomsbury USA, 2009. Print.

3. Pollan, Michael. *In Defense of Food: An Eater's Manifesto.* New York: Penguin, 2008. Print.

4. Krohn, William O. *Graded Lessons in Physiology and Hygiene: By William O. Krohn.* New York: O. Appleton, 1908. Print.

5. "Joel Salatin, America's Most Influential Farmer, Talks Big Organic and the Future of Food." *TreeHugger.* N.p., 5 Aug. 2009. Web. 08 June 2012. <http://www.treehugger.com/green-food/joel-salatin-americas-most-influential-farmer-talks-big-organic-and-the-future-of-food.html>.

Chapter 2: Why Nutrition Matters

1. J.E. Chavarro, et al. "A Prospective Study of Dairy Foods Intake and Anaovulatory Infertility." *Human Reproduction,* 22 (5): 1340-1347.

2. Boyles, Salynn. "High Doses of Vitamin D May Cut Pregnancy Risks." *WebMD.* WebMD, 4 May 2010. Web. 08 June 2012. <http://www.webmd.com/baby/news/20100504/high-doses-of-vitamin-d-may-cut-pregnancy-risk>.

3. Paul, Annie Murphy. "How the First Nine Months Shape the Rest of Your Life." *Time.* Time, 22 Sept. 2010. Web. 07 June 2012. <http://www.time.com/time/magazine/article/0,9171,2021065,00.html>.

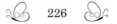

4. "Nutrition and the Epigenome," http://learn.genetics.utah.edu/content/epigenetics/nutrition/

5. Ibid.

6. Ibid.

7. Shanahan, Catherine, and Luke Shanahan. *Deep Nutrition: Why Your Genes Need Traditional Food*. Lawai, HI: Big, 2009. Print.

8. Staff, Mayo Clinic. "Male Infertility." *Mayo Clinic*. Mayo Foundation for Medical Education and Research, 09 Sept. 2011. Web. 20 June 2012. <http://www.mayoclinic.com/health/male-infertility/DS01038>.

9. Kirkey, Sharon. "Infertility Rates Rising for Canadian Couples." *Www.canada.com*. Postmedia News, 15 Feb. 2012. Web. 20 June 2012. <http://www.canada.com/health/Infertility rates rising Canadian couples/6157547/story.html>.

10. Narayan, KMV, JP Boyle, TJ Thompson, SW Sorensen, and DF Williamson. "Lifetime Risk for Diabetes Mellitus in the United States." *JAMA* 290.14 (2003): 1884-1890. Print.

11. "Cancer Statistics." *SEER Review 1975-2009 (Vintage 2009 Populations)*. N.p., n.d. Web. 20 June 2012. <http://seer.cancer.gov/csr/1975_2009_pops09/index.html>.

12. Pollan, Michael. "OPRAH AND 378 STAFFERS GO VEGAN: THE ONE-WEEK CHALLENGE." *The Oprah Winfrey Show*. CBS Television. Harpo Productions, Chicago, Illinois, 01 Feb. 2011. Television.

Chapter 3: Just Say No

1. Metcalfe, D. "Food Allergy." *Primary Care: Clinics in Office Practice* 25.4 (1998): 819-29. Print.

2. Simon, R. A. "Additive-induced Urticaria: Experience with Monosodium Glutamate (MSG)." *Journal of Nutrition* 130.4S Supplemental (2000): 1063S-066S. Print.

3. Yang, W. H., M. A. Drouin, M. Herbert, Y. Mao, and J. Karsh. "The Monosodium Glutamate Symptom Complex: Assessment in a Double-blind, Placebo-controlled, Randomized Study." *The Journal of Allergy and Clinical Immunology* Part 1 99.6 (1997): 757-62. Print.

4. Blaylock, Russell L. *Excitotoxins: The Taste That Kills.* Santa Fe, NM: Health, 1998. Print.

5. Lorden, J. F., and A. Claude. "Behavioral and Endocrinological Effects of Single Injections of Monosodium Glutamate in the Mouse." *Neurobehavioral Toxicology and Teratology* 8.5 (1986): 509-19. Print.

6. Blaylock, Russell. "Food Additives: What You Eat Can Kill You." *The Blaylock Wellness Report* 4 (Oct. 2007): 3-4. Print.

7. Blaylock, Russell L. *Excitotoxins: The Taste That Kills.* Santa Fe, NM: Health, 1998. Print.

8. Blaylock, Russell. "Food Additives: What You Eat Can Kill You." *The Blaylock Wellness Report* 4 (Oct. 2007): 3-4. Print.

9. Ohguro, H., Katsushima, H., Maruyama, I., Maeda, T., Yanagihashi, S., Metoki, T., Nakazawa, M. "A high dietary intake of sodium glutamate as flavoring (ajinomoto) causes gross changes in retinal morphology and function." *Experimental Eye Research* 75.3 (2002).: 307-15. Print.

10. Blaylock, Russell L. *Excitotoxins: The Taste That Kills.* Santa Fe, NM: Health, 1998. Print.

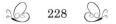

11. "Aren't The FD&C Dyes Certified To Be Safe?" *Feingold.org*. The Feingold Association of the United States, 01 June 2012. Web. 22 June 2012. <http://feingold.org/certified.php>.

12. Harris, Gardiner. "Colorless Food? We Blanch." *The New York Times*. The New York Times, 03 Apr. 2011. Web. 22 June 2012. <http://www.nytimes.com/2011/04/03/weekinreview/03harris.html?_r=3>.

13. Ibid.

14. Price, Weston A. *Nutrition and Physical Degeneration: A Comparison of Primitive and Modern Diets and Their Effects*. Oxford: Benediction Classics, 2010. Print.

15. Davis BC, Kris-Etherton PM. "Achieving optimal essential fatty acid status in vegetarians: current knowledge and practical implications." *The American Journal of Clinical Nutrition*. 78.suppl (2003):640S–6S. Print.

16. Allport, Susan. *The Queen of Fats: Why Omega-3s Were Removed from the Western Diet and What We Can Do to Replace Them*. Berkeley: University of California, 2006. Print.

17. Pollan, Michael. *The Omnivore's Dilemma: A Natural History of Four Meals*. New York: Penguin, 2006. Print.

18. Ibid.

19. Safarinejad, Mohammad Reza, Seyyed Yousof Hosseini, Farid Dadkhah, and Majid Ali Asgari. "Relationship of Omega-3 and Omega-6 Fatty Acids with Semen Characteristics, and Anti-oxidant Status of Seminal Plasma: A Comparison between Fertile and Infertile Men." *Clinical Nutrition* 29.1 (2009): 100-05. Print.

20. "Adoption of Genetically Engineered Crops in the U.S." *ERS/USDA Data*. United States Department Of Agriculture, n.d. Web. 23 June 2012. <http://www.ers.usda.gov/data/biotechcrops/>.

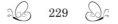

21. AFP. "Corn, Soy Crops Gain Little from Genetics." *Google News*. N.p., 14 Apr. 2009. Web. 23 June 2012. <http://www.google.com/hostednews/afp/article/ALeqM5g53DoblG25y7O5t4KPsuzYyxMd6Q>.

22. Wright, Karen. "Terminator Genes." *Discover Magazine* 1 Aug. 2003. Print.

23. Pollack, Andrew. "F.D.A. Approves Drug From Gene-Altered Goats." *The New York Times*. The New York Times, 6 Feb. 2009. Web. 23 June 2012. <http://www.nytimes.com/2009/02/07/business/07goatdrug.html?_r=2>.

24. *PHARM AND INDUSTRIAL CROPS THE NEXT WAVE OF AGRICULTURAL BIOTECHNOLOGY*. Rep. Washington, DC: Union of Concerned Scientists, 2003. Print.

25. "Say No To GMOs! - BMA Statement." *Say No To GMOs! - BMA Statement*. British Medical Association, 2009. Web. 23 June 2012. <http://www.saynotogmos.org/bma_statement.htm>.

26. Food Safety - Contaminants and Toxins. Unpublished study reviewed in J.P.F. D'Mello, CABI Publishing, 2003.

27. Malatesta M. et al. Eur J Histochem. "Fine structural analysis of pancreatic acinar cell nuclei from mice fed on GM soybean." 47: 385- 388, 2003.

28. Malatesta M. et al. "Ultrastructural morphometrical and immunocytochemical analyses of hepatocyte nuclei from mice fed on genetically modified soybean." *Cell Struct Funct.*, 27: 173-180, 2002.

29. Vecchio L. et al. "Ultrastructural analysis of testes from mice fed on genetically modified soybean." *Eur J Histochem.*, 48: 448-454, 2004.

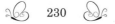

30. Prescott V.E. et al. "Transgenic expression of bean alpha-amylase inhibitor in peas results in altered structure and immunogenicity." *J Agric Food Chem.*, 53: 9023-9030, 2005.

31. "Biotechnology Consultation Note to the File BNF No 00077". Office of Food Additive Safety, Center for Food Safety and Applied Nutrition, US Food and Drug Administration, 4 September 2002.

32. Pusztai A. and Bardocz S. "GMO in animal nutrition: potential benefits and risks". *Biology of Nutrition in Growing Animals*, eds. R. Mosenthin, J. Zentek and T. Zebrowska, Elsevier Limited, pp. 513- 540, 2006.

33. Ewen S.W. and Pusztai A. "Effects of diets containing genetically modified potatoes expressing Galanthus nivalis lectin on rat small intestine". *The Lancet*, 354: 1353-1354, 1999.

34. Séralini, G.-E. et al. "New analysis of a rat feeding study with a genetically modified maize reveals signs of hepatorenal toxicity". *Arch. Environ Contam Toxicol.*, 52: 596-602, 2007.

35. Kilic A and Akay MT. "A three generation study with genetically modified Bt corn in rats: Biochemical and histopathological investigation." *Food and Chemical Toxicology*, 46: 1164-1170, 2008.

36. Finamore A et al."Intestinal and Peripheral Immune Response to MON810 Maize Ingestion in Weaning and Old Mice". *J. Agric. Food Chem.*, 56: 11533-11539, 2008.

37. Velimirov A et al."Biological effects of transgenic maize NK603x-MON810 fed in long term reproduction studies in mice". *Bundesministerium für Gesundheit, Familie und Jugend Report*, Forschungsberichte der Sektion IV Band 3/2008, Austria, 2008.

38. Malatesta M. et al."A long-term study on female mice fed on a genetically modified soybean: effects on liver ageing". *Histochem Cell Biol.*, 130: 967-977, 2008.

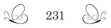

39. R. Tudisco et al. "Genetically modified soya bean in rabbit feeding: detection of DNA fragments and evaluation of metabolic effects by enzymatic analysis". *Animal Science*, 82: 193-199, 2006.

40. "A Collaborative Initiative Working to Ensure the Sustained Availability of Non-GMO Options." *The Non-GMO Project*. N.p., n.d. Web. 23 June 2012. <http://www.nongmoproject.org/>.

41. Price, Weston A., *Nutrition and Physical Degeneration: A Comparison of Primitive and Modern Diets and Their Effects*. Oxford: Benediction Classics, 2010. Print.

42. Geary, Mike. "Is Canola Oil Actually Healthy, or Is It Bad for You - Facts You Need." *The Canola Oil Marketing Deception*. N.p., n.d. Web. 22 June 2012. <http://www.truthaboutabs.com/the-canola-oil-deception.html>.

43. Chavarro Jorge E, Rich-Edwards Janet W, Rosner Bernard A and Willett Walter C (2007-01). "Dietary fatty acid intakes and the risk of ovulatory infertility". *American Journal of Clinical Nutrition* **85** (1): 231–237.

44. "Corn Oil." *National Nutrient Database for Standard Reference Release 24*. USDA, n.d. Web. 20 June 2012.

45. Lands, William E. M. *Fish, Omega 3 and Human Health*. Champaign, IL: AOCS, 2005. Print.

46. Pew Campaign on Human Health and Industrial Farming. "Human Health and Industrial Farming: The Basics." *Pew Health Group*. Pew Charitable Trusts, 16 Mar. 2010. Web. 22 June 2012. <http://www.pewhealth.org/reports-analysis/issue-briefs/human-health-and-industrial-farming-the-basics-85899391511>.

47. Pew Commission on Industrial Farm Animal Production. *Putting Meat on The Table: Industrial Farm Animal Production in America*. Rep. N.p.: Pew Charitable Trusts, 2009. Print.

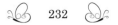

48. Pew Campaign on Human Health and Industrial Farming. "Human Health and Industrial Farming: The Basics." *Pew Health Group*. Pew Charitable Trusts, 16 Mar. 2010. Web. 22 June 2012. <http://www.pewhealth.org/reports-analysis/issue-briefs/human-health-and-industrial-farming-the-basics-85899391511>.

49. Ibid.

50. Pollan, Michael. *The Omnivore's Dilemma: A Natural History of Four Meals*. New York: Penguin, 2006. Print.

51. Ibid.

52. Michaels, Ann Marie. "Will the Real California Happy Cows Please Stand Up?" *CHEESESLAVE*. N.p., 28 Mar. 2011. Web. 30 June 2012. <http://www.cheeseslave.com/will-the-real-california-happy-cows-please-stand-up/>.

53. Woodford, K. B. *Devil in the Milk: Illness, Health and Politics of A1 and A2 Milk*. White River Junction, VT: Chelsea Green Pub., 2009. Print.

54. Fallon, Sally, Mary G. Enig, Kim Murray, and Marion Dearth. *Nourishing Traditions: The Cookbook That Challenges Politically Correct Nutrition and the Diet Dictocrats*. Washington, DC: NewTrends Pub., 2001. Print.

55. Enig, Mary. "Milk Homogenization & Heart Disease." *Wise Traditions in Food, Farming and the Healing Arts* Summer (2003). Print.

56. Fallon, Sally, Mary G. Enig, Kim Murray, and Marion Dearth. *Nourishing Traditions: The Cookbook That Challenges Politically Correct Nutrition and the Diet Dictocrats*. Washington, DC: NewTrends Pub., 2001. Print.

57. Dalton, Joseph P. "Antibiotic Residue Avoidance in Milk and Dairy Beef." *Progressive Dairyman Magazine*. N.p., n.d. Web. 22 June 2012. <http://www.progressivedairy.com/index.php?option=com_content>.

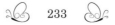

58. Epstein, S. S. "Potential public health hazards of biosynthetic milk hormones." *International Journal of Health Services*, 20:73-84, 1990. Print.

59. Kristof, Nicholas D. "Arsenic In Our Chicken?" *The New York Times*. The New York Times, 05 Apr. 2012. Web. 22 June 2012. <http://www.nytimes.com/2012/04/05/opinion/kristof-arsenic-in-our-chicken.html>.

60. Vallaeys, Charlotte. *Scrambled Eggs: Separating Factory Farm Egg Production from Authentic Organic Agriculture*. Rep. Cornucopia: Cornucopia Institute, 2010. Print.

61. Ibid.

62. Ibid.

63. Megan, Manlove. "Route to Obesity Passes through Tongue." *Penn State Live*. Penn State University, 28 Nov. 2008. Web. 23 June 2012. <http://live.psu.edu/story/36294>.

64. "Sugar and Sweeteners: Recommended Data." *ERS/USDA Briefing Room -*. United States Department Of Agriculture, n.d. Web. 23 June 2012. <http://www.ers.usda.gov/briefing/sugar/data.htm>.

65. Sanchez, A., et al. "Role of Sugars in Human Neutrophilic Phagocytosis", *American Journal of Clinical Nutrition*. Nov 1973;261:1180_1184. Bernstein, J., al. "Depression of Lymphocyte Transformation Following Oral Glucose Ingestion." *American Journal of Clinical Nutrition*.1997;30:613

66. Goldman, J., et al. "Behavioral Effects of Sucrose on Preschool Children." *Journal of Abnormal Child Psychology*.1986;14(4):565_577

67. Scanto, S. and Yudkin, J. "The Effect of Dietary Sucrose on Blood Lipids, Serum Insulin, Platelet Adhesiveness and Body Weight in Human Volunteers", *Postgraduate Medicine Journal*. 1969;45:602_607

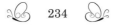

68. Albrink, M. and Ullrich I. H. "Interaction of Dietary Sucrose and Fiber on Serum Lipids in Healthy Young Men Fed High Carbohydrate Diets". *American Journal of Clinical Nutrition.* 1986;43:419

69. Reiser, S. "Effects of Dietary Sugars on Metabolic Risk Factors Associated with Heart Disease". *Nutritional Health.* 1985;203_216

70. Lewis, G. F. and Steiner, G. "Acute Effects of Insulin in the Control of Vldl Production in Humans. Implications for The insulin-resistant State". *Diabetes Care.* 1996 Apr;19(4):390-3 R. Pamplona, M. .J., et al. Mechanisms of Glycation in Atherogenesis. Medical Hypotheses. 1990;40:174-181

71. Takahashi, E., Tohoku University School of Medicine, *Wholistic Health Digest.* October 1982:41:00

72. Quillin, Patrick, "Cancer's Sweet Tooth," *Nutrition Science News.* Ap 2000 Rothkopf, M.. *Nutrition.* July/Aug 1990;6(4)

73. Michaud, D. "Dietary Sugar, Glycemic Load, and Pancreatic Cancer Risk in a Prospective Study." *Journal of the National Cancer Institute.* Sep 4, 2002 ;94(17):1293-300

74. Moerman, C. J., et al. "Dietary Sugar Intake in the Etiology of Biliary Tract Cancer". *International Journal of Epidemiology.* Ap 1993.2(2):207-214.

75. The Edell Health Letter. Sept 1991;7:1

76. De Stefani, E."Dietary Sugar and Lung Cancer: a Case control Study in Uruguay." *Nutrition and Cancer.* 1998;31(2):132_7

77. Cornee, J., et al. "A Case-control Study of Gastric Cancer and Nutritional Factors in Marseille, France". *European Journal of Epidemiology* 11 (1995):55-65

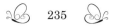

78. Yudkin, J. "Metabolic Changes Induced by Sugar in Relation to Coronary Heart Disease and Diabetes". *Nutrition and Health.* 1987;5(1-2):5-8

79. Yudkin, J and Eisa, O. "Dietary Sucrose and Oestradiol Concentration in Young Men". *Annals of Nutrition and Metabolism.* 1988:32(2):53-55

80. The Edell Health Letter. Sept 1991;7:1

81. Gardner, L. and Reiser, S. "Effects of Dietary Carbohydrate on Fasting Levels of Human Growth Hormone and Cortisol". *Proceedings of the Society for Experimental Biology and Medicine.* 1982;169:36_40

82. Hogeveen, Kevin N., Patrice Cousin, Michel Pugeat, Didier Dewailly, Benoît Soudan, and Geoffrey L. Hammond. "Human Sex Hormone–binding Globulin Variants Associated with Hyperandrogenism and Ovarian Dysfunction." *Journal of Clinical Investigation* 109.7 (2002): 973-81. Print.

83. "Joel Salatin January 27, 2010." *Underground Wellness.* Blog Talk Radio. 27 Jan. 2010. Radio.

84. Howard, Albert. *The Soil and Health: A Study of Organic Agriculture.* Lexington: University of Kentucky, 2006. Print.

85. Kimbrell, Andrew. *The Fatal Harvest Reader: The Tragedy of Industrial Agriculture.* Washington: Published by the Foundation for Deep Ecology in Collaboration with Island, 2002. Print.

86. Philpott, Tom. "A Debate about Soil, Organics, And nutrition." *Grist.* N.p., 13 Aug. 2009. Web. 23 June 2012. <http://grist.org/article/2009-08-13-debate-soil-organics-nutrition/>.

87. Halwell, Brian. *Still No Free Lunch: Nutrient Levels in U.S. Food Supply Eroded by Pursuit of High Yields.* Rep. Vol. September. Boulder: Organic Center, 2007. Print.

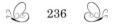

88. Jean, Nancy C. "Researchers Find Possible Environmental Causes for Alzheimer's, Diabetes." *JAD - Press Releases*. Journal of Alzheimer's Disease, 6 July 2009. Web. 23 June 2012. <http://www.j-alz.com/press/2009/20090706.html>.

89. "Food Storage And Vitamin Losses." *Food Storage And Vitamin Losses*. N.p., n.d. Web. 23 June 2012. <http://www.vitamin-deficiency-today.com/food-storage.html>.

90. Tabrizian, Igor. *Nutrition: The Good, the Bad and the Politics*. [Yokine, W.A.]: NRS Publications, 2006. Print.

Chapter 4: What to Eat Instead

1. Pollan, Michael. "BEFORE YOU GROCERY SHOP AGAIN: FOOD 101 WITH MICHAEL POLLAN" *The Oprah Winfrey Show*. CBS Television. Harpo Productions, Chicago, Illinois, 27 Jan. 2011. Television.

2. Michaelis, Kristen. "Guest Post: Joel Salatin on Why Local Food Is More Expensive." *Food Renegade*. N.p., 8 Apr. 2009. Web. 23 June 2012. <http://www.foodrenegade.com/guest-post-joel-salatin-on-why-local-food-is-more-expensive/>

3. Fallon, Sally. "Broth Is Beautiful." - *Weston A Price Foundation*. N.p., 1 Jan. 2000. Web. 23 June 2012. <http://www.westonaprice.org/food-features/broth-is-beautiful>.

4. Pitchford, Paul. *Healing with Whole Foods: Asian Traditions and Modern Nutrition*. Berkeley, CA: North Atlantic, 2002. Print.

5. Forge, Arabella, and Genna Campton. *Frugavore: How to Grow Organic, Buy Local, Waste Nothing, and Eat Well*. New York: Skyhorse Pub., 2011. Print.

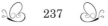

6. Fallon, Sally. "Broth Is Beautiful." - *Weston A Price Foundation*. N.p., 1 Jan. 2000. Web. 23 June 2012. <http://www.westonaprice.org/food-features/broth-is-beautiful>.

7. Daniel, Kaayla. "Why Broth Is Beautiful: Essential Roles for Proline, Glycine and Gelatin." *Weston A Price Foundation*. N.p., 18 June 2003. Web. 24 June 2012. <http://www.westonaprice.org/food-features/why-broth-is-beautiful>.

8. Robinson, Jo. "What You Need to Know About The Beef You Eat." *Mother Earth News*. N.p., Feb. 2008. Web. 24 June 2012. <http://www.motherearthnews.com/Sustainable-Farming/2008-02-01/What-You-Need-to-Know-About-the-Beef-You-Eat.aspx>.

9. Belury, M.A. "Inhibition of carcinogenesis by conjugated linoleic acid: Potential mechanisms of action". *Journal of Nutrition* 132 (10): 2995–2998, 2002.

10. Amarù DL, Field CJ. "Conjugated Linoleic Acid Decreases MCF-7 Human Breast Cancer Cell Growth and Insulin-Like Growth Factor-1 Receptor Levels". *Lipids* 26 (5): 449–58, 2009.

11. Lee Y, Thompson JT, de Lera AR, Vanden Heuvel JP. "Isomer-specific effects of conjugated linoleic acid on gene expression in RAW 264.7". *Journal of Nutritional Biochemestry* 26 (11): 848–59, 2008.

12. Coakley M, Banni S, Johnson MC, Mills S, Devery R, Fitzgerald G, Paul Ross R, Stanton C. "Inhibitory Effect of Conjugated alpha-Linolenic Acid from Bifidobacteria of Intestinal Origin on SW480 Cancer Cells". *Lipids* **44** (3): 249–56, 2009.

13. Ip C, Scimeca JA, Thompson HJ. "Conjugated linoleic acid. A powerful anticarcinogen from animal fat sources". *Cancer* 74 (3): 1050–4, 1994.

14. Kritchevsky D. "Antimutagenic and some other effects of conjugated linoleic acid". *British Journal of Nutrition*. 83 (5): 459–65, 2000.

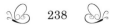

15. Pariza MW, Park Y, Cook ME. "The biologically active isomers of conjugated linoleic acid". *Prog Lipid Res.* 40 (4): 283–98, 2001.

16. Bhattacharya A., Banu J., Rahman M., Causey J., Fernandes G. "Biological effects of conjugated linoleic acids in health and disease". *J Nutr Biochem.* 17 (12): 789–810, 2006.

17. Donnelly C, Olsen AM, Lewis LD, Eisenberg BL, Eastman A, Kinlaw WB. "Conjugated Linoleic Acid (CLA) inhibits expression of the Spot 14 (THRSP) and fatty acid synthase genes and impairs the growth of human breast cancer and liposarcoma cells". *Nutr Cancer.* 61 (1): 114–22, 2009.

18. Islam MA, Kim YS, Jang WJ, Lee SM, Kim HG, Kim SY, Kim JO, Ha YL. "A mixture of trans, trans conjugated linoleic acid induces apoptosis in MCF-7 human breast cancer cells with reciprocal expression of Bax and Bcl-2". *J Agric Food Chem* (Korea) 56 (14): 5970–6, 2008.

19. Kelley NS, Hubbard NE, Erickson KL. "Conjugated linoleic acid isomers and cancer". *J Nutr* (UC Davis, Ca, USA) 137 (12): 2599–607, 2007.

20. Fite A, Goua M, Wahle KW, Schofield AC, Hutcheon AW, Heys SD. "Potentiation of the anti-tumour effect of docetaxel by conjugated linoleic acids (CLAs) in breast cancer cells in vitro". *Prostaglandins Leukot Essent Fatty Acids.* (Scotland, UK) 77 (2): 87–96, 2007.

21. Tricon S, Burdge GC, Kew S et al. "Opposing effects of cis-9,trans-11 and trans-10,cis-12 conjugated linoleic acid on blood lipids in healthy humans". *American Journal of Clinical Noutrition.* 80 (3): 614–20, 2004.

22. Zulet MA, Marti A, Parra MD, Martínez JA . "Inflammation and conjugated linoleic acid: mechanisms of action and implications for human health". *J. Physiol. Biochem.* 61 (3): 483–94, 2005.

23. Whigham L et al. "Efficacy of conjugated linoleic acid for reducing fat mass:a meta-analysis in humans". *American Journal of Clinical Nutrition.* 85 (5): 1203–11, 2007.

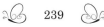

24. Bassaganya-Riera, J; Reynolds, K; Martino-Catt, S; Cui, Y; Henni-ghausen, L; Gonzalez, F; Rohrer, J; Benninghoff, AU et al. . "Activation of PPAR gamma and delta by conjugated linoleic acid mediates protection from experimental inflammatory bowel disease". *Gastroenterology* 127 (3): 777–91, 2004.

25. "Researchers Discover Novel Therapy for Chron's Disease." *Virginia Bioinformatics Institute.* Virginia Tech, 16 Mar. 2012. Web. 22 June 2012. <http://www.vbi.vt.edu/marketing_and_communications/press_releas-es_view/researchers_discover_novel_therapy_for_crohns_disease>.

26. Pollan, Michael. *The Omnivore's Dilemma: A Natural History of Four Meals.* New York: Penguin, 2006. Print.

27. "Soil Health." *Organic Trade Association.* Organic Trade Association, n.d. Web. 20 June 2012. <www.ota.com/organic/benefits/soil.html>.

28. "The Chicken and Egg Page." *Mother Earth News.* Mother Earth News, 29 Mar. 2007. Web. 24 June 2012. <http://www.motherearthnews.com/eggs.aspx>.

29. Vallaeys, Charlotte. *Scrambled Eggs: Separating Factory Farm Egg Production from Authentic Organic Agriculture.* Rep. Cornucopia: Cor-nucopia Institute, 2010. Print.

30. "Mercury in Stream Ecosystems." *National Water Quality Assess-ment Program.* United States Geological Survey, n.d. Web. 24 June 2012. <http://water.usgs.gov/nawqa/mercury/>.

31. Price, Weston A. Nutrition and Physical Degeneration: A Compari-son of Primitive and Modern Diets and Their Effects. Oxford: Benedic-tion Classics, 2010. Print.

32. Fallon, Sally. "Nourished Magazine." *Ask Sally Fallon: Milk :: Cho-lesterol :: Mercury in Seafood :: Constipation.* Nourished Magazine, 1 July 2008. Web. 24 June 2012. <http://nourishedmagazine.com.au/blog/ar-ticles/milk-cholesterol-mercury-in-seafood>.

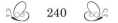

33. Rowland, I. R., J. M. Davies, and J. G. Evans. "Tissue Content of Mercury in Rats given Methylmercuric Chloride Orally: Influence of Intestinal Flora." *Arch. Environ. Health* 35.3 (1980): 155-60. Print.

34. Planck, Nina. *Real Food for Mother and Baby: The Fertility Diet, Eating for Two, and Baby's First Foods.* New York: Bloomsbury USA, 2009. Print.

35. "Collection of Coconut Sap." *Wilderness Family Naturals.* Wilderness Family Naturals, n.d. Web. 24 June 2012. <http://www.wildernessfamilynaturals.com/collection-of-coconut-sap.php>.

36. Arnold, David. "India and the Early Discourse on Beriberi." *National Center for Biotechnology Information.* U.S. National Library of Medicine, 29 Dec. 0005. Web. 25 June 2012. <http://www.ncbi.nlm.nih.gov/pmc/articles/PMC2889456/>.

37. Rajakumar, K. "Pellagra in the United States: A Historical Perspective". *Southern Medical Journal* 98 (3): 272–277, 2000.

38. Rothman, KJ, Moore LL, Singer MR, Et Al. "Teratogenicity of High Vitamin A Intake" *New England Journal of Medicine* 1995;333:1369-1373. Print.

39. Miyake, K., T. Tanaka, and P. L. McNeil. "Disruption-Induced Mucus Secretion: Repair and Protection." *PLoS Biology* 4.9 (2006): E276. Print.

40. Freed, David LJ. "Do Dietary Lectins Cause Disease?" *British Medical Journal* 318.7190 (1999): 1023-024. Print.

41. Gregor, J. L. "Nondigestible Carbohydrates and Mineral Bioavailability." *Journal of Nutrition* 129.7 (1999): 1434S-435s. Print.

42. Mellanby, M., and C. L. Pattison. "Remarks on the influence of a cereal-free diet rich in Vitamin D and calcium on dental caries in children." *British Medical Journal* 1.3715 (1932): 507-10. Print.

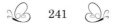

43. Sandberg, A.-S., and U. Svanberg. "Phytate Hydrolysis by Phytase in Cereals; Effects on In Vitro Estimation of Iron Availability." *Journal of Food Science* 56.5 (1991): 1330-333. Print.

44. Schober, Tilman J., Scott R. Bean, and Daniel L. Boyle. "Gluten-Free Sorghum Bread Improved by Sourdough Fermentation: Biochemical, Rheological, and Microstructural Background." *Journal of Agricultural and Food Chemistry* 55.13 (2007): 5137-146. Print.

45. Sapirstein, H.d., P. David, K.r. Preston, and J.e. Dexter. "Durum Wheat Breadmaking Quality: Effects of Gluten Strength, Protein Composition, Semolina Particle Size and Fermentation Time." *Journal of Cereal Science* 45.2 (2007): 150-61. Print.

46. Khetarpaul, Neelam, and B.M. Chauhan. "Effects of Germination and Pure Culture Fermentation by Yeasts and Lactobacilli on Phytic Acid and Polyphenol Content of Pearl Millet." *Journal of Food Science* 55.4 (1990): 1180. Print.

47. "Wheat, sprouted." *National Nutrient Database for Standard Reference Release 24.* USDA, n.d. Web. 20 June 2012.

Chapter 5: Taking Care of the Gut

1. Blakeslee, Sandra. "Complex and Hidden Brain in Gut Makes Stomachaches and Butterflies." *The New York Times* 23 Jan. 1996. Print.

2. Gershon, Michael D. *The Second Brain: A Groundbreaking New Understanding of Nervous Disorders of the Stomach and Intestine.* New York, NY: HarperPerennial, 1999. Print.

3. Fallon, Sally, and Mary Enig. "The Long Hollow Tube: A Primer on the Digestive System." *Weston A Price Foundation.* Weston A Price Foundation, 23 Sept. 2004. Web. 25 June 2012. <http://www.westonaprice.org/digestive-disorders/primer-digestive-system>.

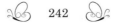

4. Campbell-McBride, Natasha. *Gut and Psychology Syndrome: Natural Treatment for Autism, Dyspraxia, A.D.D., Dyslexia, A.D.H.D., Depression, Schizophrenia*. Cambridge, U.K.: Medinform Pub., 2010. Print.

5. Ibid.

6. Lewis SJ, Heaton KW. "Stool form scale as a useful guide to intestinal transit time". *Scand. J. Gastroenterol.* 32 (9): 920–4, 1997.

7. Pop, Mihai. "We Are What We Eat: How the Diet of Infants Affects Their Gut Microbiome." *Genome Biology* 13.4 (2012): 152. Print.

8. Dethlefsena, Les, and David A. Relmana. "Incomplete Recovery and Individualized Responses of the Human Distal Gut Microbiota to Repeated Antibiotic Perturbation." *Proceedings of the National Academy of Sciences of the United States of America* 108.Supplement 1 (2011): 4554-561. Print.

9. Jakobsson, Hedvig E., Cecilia Jernberg, Anders F. Andersson, Maria Sjölund-Karlsson, Janet K. Jansson, and Lars Engstrand. "Short-Term Antibiotic Treatment Has Differing Long-Term Impacts on the Human Throat and Gut Microbiome." Ed. Adam J. Ratner. *PLoS ONE* 5.3 (2010): E9836. Print.

10. Sjölund, Maria, Karin Wreiber, Dan I. Andersson, Martin J. Blaser, and Lars Engstrand. "Long-Term Persistence of Resistant Enterococcus Species after Antibiotics To Eradicate Helicobacter Pylori." *Annals of Internal Medicine* 139.6 (2003): 483-87. Print.

11. Crook, William G. *The Yeast Connection: A Medical Breakthrough*. New York: Vintage, 1986. Print.

12. Rowland, I. R., J. M. Davies, and J. G. Evans. "Tissue Content of Mercury in Rats given Methylmercuric Chloride Orally: Influence of Intestinal Flora." *Arch. Environ. Health* 35.3 (1980): 155-60. Print.

13. Friberg, Lars, and Ernst Hammarström. "THE ACTION OF FREE AVAILABLE CHLORINE ON BACTERIA AND BACTERIAL VIRUSES." *Acta Pathologica Microbiologica Scandinavica* 38.2 (1956): 127-34. Print.

14. Gorbach, S. L. "Estrogens, Breast Cancer, and Intestinal Flora." *Clinical Infectious Diseases* 6.Supplement 1 (1984): S85-90. Print.

15. Ouwehand, Arthur, and Elaine E. Vaughan. *Gastrointestinal Microbiology*. New York: Taylor & Francis, 2006. Print.

16. Price, Weston A. *Nutrition and Physical Degeneration: A Comparison of Primitive and Modern Diets and Their Effects*. Oxford: Benediction Classics, 2010. Print.

17. Ljungh, Åsa, and Torkel Wadström. *Lactobacillus Molecular Biology: From Genomics to Probiotics*. Norfolk, UK: Caister Academic, 2009. Print.

Chapter 6: Eating For Fertility and Pregnancy

1. Price, Weston A. *Nutrition and Physical Degeneration: A Comparison of Primitive and Modern Diets and Their Effects*. Oxford: Benediction Classics, 2010. Print.

2. Masterjohn, Chris. "Vitamins for Fetal Development: Conception to Birth." *Weston A Price Foundation*. Weston A Price Foundation, 22 Mar. 2009. Web. 25 June 2012. <http://www.westonaprice.org/childrens-health/vitamins-for-fetal-development-conception-to-birth>.

3. Dean, Carolyn. *The Magnesium Miracle: Discover the Essential Nutrient That Will Lower Therisk of Heart Disease, Prevent Stroke and Obesity, Treat Diabetes, and Improve Mood and Memory*. New York: Ballantine, 2007. Print.

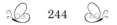

4. Golf SW, Bender S, Grüttner J. "On the significance of magnesium in extreme physical stress". *Cardiovascular drugs and therapy / sponsored by the International Society of Cardiovascular Pharmacotherapy.* 12 2. Supplement 2 (1998): 197–202.

5. Muneyyirci-Delale, Ozgul, Bella T. Altura, Burton Altura, Madar Dalloul, and Vijaya L. Nacharaju. "Serum Ionized Magnesium and Calcium in Women after Menopause: Inverse Relation of Estrogen with Ionized Magnesium." *Elsevier* 71.5 (1999): 869-72. Print.

6. Abraham, G. E., M. M. Lubran, and U. D. Schwartz. "Effect of Vitamin B-6 on Plasma and Red Blood Cell Magnesium Levels in Premenopausal Women." *Annals of Clinical and Laboratory Science* 4.11 (1981): 333-36. Print.

7. Eliakim, R., Abulafia, O., & Sherer, D. M. (2000). "Hyperemesis gravidarum: A current review". *American Journal of Perinatology* **17** (4): 207–218.

8. Wolverton, George M. "The Magic of B Complex B12." *The Magic of B Complex B12.* The Evergreene Medical Centre, n.d. Web. 26 June 2012. <http://www.evergreenmedicalcentre.com/Articles/magic_B_complex_B12.html>.

9. Hardwick, L. L., M. R. Jones, N. Brautbar, and D. B. Lee. "Magnesium Absorption: Mechanisms and the Influence of Vitamin D, Calcium and Phosphate." *Journal of Nutrition* 121.1 (1991): 13-23. Print.

10. Waring, R. H. "Absorption of Magnesium Sulfate across the Skin." *Magnesium Online Library.* The Magnesium Website, 10 Jan. 2004. Web. 26 June 2012. <http://www.mgwater.com/transdermal.shtml>.

11. Brewer, Gail Sforza., and Thomas H. Brewer. *The Brewer Medical Diet for Normal and High-risk Pregnancy: A Leading Obstetrician's Guide to Every Stage of Pregnancy.* New York: Simon and Schuster, 1983. Print.

12. Jones, Joy. "Frequently Asked Questions." *The Dr. Brewer Pregnancy Diet*. N.p., n.d. Web. 26 June 2012. <http://www.drbrewerpregnancydiet.com/id13.html>.

13. Roe DA. "Current etiologies and cutaneous signs of vitamin deficiencies." In: Roe DA, ed. *Nutrition and the skin. Contemporary issues in clinical nutrition*. New York: Alan R Liss Inc, 1986:81–98. Print.

14. Nagata, Chisato, Kozue Nakamura, Keiko Wada, Shino Oba, Makoto Hayashi, Noriyuki Takeda, and Keigo Yasuda. "Association of Dietary Fat, Vegetables and Antioxidant Micronutrients with Skin Ageing in Japanese Women." *British Journal of Nutrition* 103.10 (2010): 1493-498. Print.

15. Segger, Dorte, Andreas Matthies, and Tom Saldeen. "Supplementation with Eskimo® Skin Care Improves Skin Elasticity in Women. A Pilot Study." *Journal of Dermatological Treatment* 19.5 (2008): 279-83. Print.

16. Palombo, P., G. Fabrizi, V. Ruocco, E. Ruocco, J. Fluhr, R. Roberts, and P. Morganti. "Beneficial Long-Term Effects of Combined Oral/Topical Antioxidant Treatment with the Carotenoids Lutein and Zeaxanthin on Human Skin: A Double-Blind, Placebo-Controlled Study." *Skin Pharmacology and Physiology* 20.4 (2007): 199-210. Print.

17. Rhemus, Wingfield, Shireen Guide, Annie Chiu, Susan Chon, Shawn Talbot, Dale Kern, and Alexa Kimball. *A Randomized Placebo-Controlled Pilot Trial to Assess the Effects of 5 Different Food Supplements on Skin*. Rep. Stanford: Stanford University, 2012. Print.

Chapter 7: Nutritional Myth-Busting

1. Mente, A., L. De Koning, H. S. Shannon, and S. S. Anand. "A Systematic Review of the Evidence Supporting a Causal Link Between Dietary Factors and Coronary Heart Disease." *Archives of Internal Medicine* 169.7 (2009): 659-69. Print.

2. Siri-Tarino, P. W., Q. Sun, F. B. Hu, and R. M. Krauss. "Meta-analysis of Prospective Cohort Studies Evaluating the Association of Saturated Fat with Cardiovascular Disease." *American Journal of Clinical Nutrition* 91.3 (2010): 535-46. Print.

3. Bloomer, Allsion. "What Does Saturated Fat Cause? Arguments." *The Boston Globe* 24 Feb. 2010. Print.

4. Campbell-McBride, Natasha. "Cholesterol: Friend Or Foe?" *Weston A Price Foundation*. Weston A Price Foundation, 4 May 2008. Web. 26 June 2012. <http://www.westonaprice.org/know-your-fats/cholesterol-friend-or-foe>.

5. Scholl TO. Iron status during pregnancy: setting the stage for mother and infant. *Am J Clin Nutr.* 2005;81(5):1218S-1222.

6. Planck, Nina. *Real Food for Mother and Baby: The Fertility Diet, Eating for Two, and Baby's First Foods.* New York: Bloomsbury USA, 2009. Print.

7. Steer P, Alam MA, Wadsworth J, Welch A. "Relation between maternal haemoglobin concentration and birth weight in different ethnic groups." *British Medical Journal* 310(1995):489-91. Print.

8. "Listeria and Pregnancy." *American Pregnancy Association*. American Pregnancy Association, June 2011. Web. 26 June 2012. <http://www.americanpregnancy.org/pregnancycomplications/listeria.html>.

9. Salatin, Joel. "Pastured Poultry: The Polyface Farm Model." *Weston A Price Foundation*. Weston A Price Foundation, 30 Sept. 2002. Web. 26

June 2012. <http://www.westonaprice.org/farm-a-ranch/pastured-poul-try-polyface-farm>.

10. Kelly, Yvonne. "Light Drinking during Pregnancy: Still No Increased Risk for Socioemotional Difficulties or Cognitive Deficits at 5 years of Age." *Journal of Epidemiology and Community Health* 66.1 (2012): 41-48. Print.

11. "Danish Studies Suggest Low and Moderate Drinking in Early Pregnancy Has No Adverse Effects on Children Aged Five." *British Journal of Obstetrics and Gynecology*. BJOG, 20 June 2012. Web. 26 June 2012. <http://www.bjog.org/details/news/2085661/Danish_studies_suggest_low_and_moderate_drinking_in_early_pregnancy_has_no_adver.html>.

12. Patrick, Clarence Hodges. *Alcohol, Culture, and Society.* Durham, N. C.: Duke Univ., 1952. Print.

13. Dasgupta, Amitava. *The Science of Drinking: How Alcohol Affects Your Body and Mind.* Lanham, MD: Rowman & Littlefield, 2011. Print.

14. "'Oldest Known Wine-making Facility' Found in Armenia." *BBC News*. BBC, 01 Nov. 2011. Web. 26 June 2012. <http://www.bbc.co.uk/news/world-europe-12158341>.

Chapter 8: Beyond Nutrition: Exploring Alternative Treatments for Fertility & Pregnancy

1. Jason, et al., "Incidence of Adverse Drug Reactions in Hospitalized Patients," *Journal of the American Medical Association* 279.15 (1998): 1200-05. Print.

2. Ibid.

3. Thomas, E.J., D.M. Studdert, H.R. Burstin, E.J. Orav, T. Zeena, E.J. Williams, K.M. Howard, P.C. Weiler, and T.A. Brennan. "Incidence and

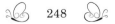

Types of Adverse Events and Negligent Care in Utah and Colorado." Medical Care 38.3 (2000):261-71. *Print.*

4. Xakellis, G. C., et al., "Cost of Pressure Ulcer Prevention in Long Term Care." Journal of the American Geriatri*cs Society 43.5 (1995): 496-501. Print.*

5. Forth Decennial International Conference on Nosocomial and Healthcare-Associated Infections, Morbidity and Mortality Weekly Report (MMWR), February 25, 2000, Vol. 49, No. 7, p. 138. Print.

6. Greene Burger S, Kayser-Jones J, Prince Bell J. "Malnutrition and Dehydration in Nursing Homes:Key Issues in Prevention and Treatment," National Citizens' *Coalition for Nursing Home Reform. June 2000. Print.*

7. Starfield B., "Is US health really the best in the world?" Journal of the American Medical Association. 284.4 (2000):483-5. Star*field B., "Deficiencies in US medical care." Journal of the American Medical Association. 284.17 (2000):2184-5.*

8. Calculations detailed in "Unnecessary Surgery" section, from two sources: (1) http://hcup.ahrq.gov/HCUPnet.asp and (2) US Congressional House Subcommittee Oversight Investigation. Cost and Quality of Health Care: Unnecessary Surgery. Washington, DC: Government Printing Office, 1976

9. "Agency for Healthcare Research and Quality (AHRQ) Home." Agency for Healthcare Research and Quality (AHRQ) Home. N.*p., n.d. Web. 26 June 2012. <http://www.ahrq.gov/>.*

10. "Leading Causes of Death." *Centers for Disease Control and Prevention.* Centers for Disease Control and Prevention, 27 Jan. 2012. Web. 26 June 2012. <http://www.cdc.gov/nchs/fastats/lcod.htm>.

11. Adams, Kelly M. "Status of Nutrition Education in Medical Schools." *American Journal of Clinical Nutrition* 83.4 (2006): 941S-44S. Print.

12. Rowley, Robert. "The 25 Most Common Diagnoses." *Electronic Health Records*. Electronic Health Records, 9 Feb. 2011. Web. 27 June 2012. <http://www.practicefusion.com/ehrbloggers/2011/02/25-most-common-diagnoses.html>.

13. Price, Weston A. *Nutrition and Physical Degeneration: A Comparison of Primitive and Modern Diets and Their Effects*. Oxford: Benediction Classics, 2010. Print.

14. Barnes PM, Powell-Griner E, McFann K, Nahin RL. "Complementary and alternative medicine use among adults: United States, 2002". *Advance Data*. 343 (2004): 1–19.

15. Eisenberg, D. M. "Trends in Alternative Medicine Use in the United States, 1990–1997: Results of a Follow-up National Survey." *Journal of the American Medical Association* 280.18 (1998): 1569-575. Print.

16. Ibid.

17. Smith, J. F. "The Use of Complementary and Alternative Fertility Treatment in Couples Seeking Fertility Care: Data from a Prospective Cohort in the United States." *Fertility and Sterility* 93.7 (2010): 2169-174. Print.

18. Manheimer, E., G. Zhang, L. Udoff, A. Haramati, P. Langenberg, B.M. Berman, and L.M. Bouter. "Effects of Acupuncture on Rates of Pregnancy and Live Birth Among Women Undergoing In Vitro Fertilization: Systematic Review and Meta-Analysis." *Obstetric Anesthesia Digest* 28.3 (2008): 150. Print.

19. Domar, Alice D., Irene Meshay, Joseph Kelliher, Michael Alper, and R. Douglas Powers. "The Impact of Acupuncture on in Vitro Fertilization Outcome." *Fertility and Sterility* 91.3 (2009): 723-26. Print.

20. Jones, Joie P., and Young K. Bae. "Ultrasonic Visualization and Stimulation of Classical Oriental Acupuncture Points." *Medical Acupuncture* 15.2 (2004): 24-26. Print.

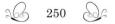

21. Chang, R. "Role of Acupuncture in the Treatment of Female Infertility." *Fertility and Sterility* 78.6 (2002): 1149-153. Print.

22. Conis, Elena. "Acupuncture for Fertility: Doctors Say, 'Why Not?'" *Los Angeles Times*. Los Angeles Times, 04 July 2005. Web. 27 June 2012. <http://articles.latimes.com/2005/jul/04/health/he-acupunc4>.

23. "Acupuncture: A Cure for Infertility? | Fox News." *Fox News*. FOX News Network, 26 Apr. 2005. Web. 27 June 2012. <http://www.foxnews.com/story/0,2933,154472,00.html>.

24. A Spine Tingling Affair." *The Monterey County Herald* Mar. 1998, sec. D: 1. Print.

25. Behrendt, M. "Insult, Interference and Infertility: An Overview of Chiropractic Research." *Journal of Vertebral Subluxation Research* May (2003): 1-8. Print.

26. Lee, H., Y. Elsayed, and J. Gould. "Population Trends in Cesarean Delivery for Breech Presentation in the United States, 1997-2003." *American Journal of Obstetrics and Gynecology* 199.1 (2008): 59.e1-9.e8. Print.

27. Whitehead, Nicole. "For Many Pregnant Moms, Webster Technique Is the Key to a Safer Birth." *Pathways to Family Wellness* Summer 2007. Web.

28. Ibid.

29. Hemilä, H; Chalker E, Douglas B. "Vitamin C for preventing and treating the common cold". *Cochrane Database of Systematic Reviews* 3.2 (2000): CD000980. Print.

30. *Infant Mortality Rate (Infant Deaths per 1,000 Live Births)*. Rep. : Population Reference Bureau. *Population Reference Bureau*. Web. 25 July 2012.

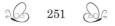

31. "The World Fact Book." *Central Intelligence Agency.* United States of America, n.d. Web. 27 June 2012. <https://www.cia.gov/library/publications/the-world-factbook/>.

32. Shanley, Laura. "Changing Fear/Tension/Pain into Faith/Relaxation/ Pleasure." *Unassisted Childbirth.* N.p., n.d. Web. 27 June 2012. <http:// www.unassistedchildbirth.com/joy-be-inspired/changing-feartension-pain-into-faithrelaxationpleasure/>.

Chapter 9: Breastfeeding and Homemade Formulas

1. Planck, Nina. *Real Food for Mother and Baby: The Fertility Diet, Eating for Two, and Baby's First Foods.* New York: Bloomsbury USA, 2009. Print.

2. Fomon, Samuel J. "Infant Feeding in the 20th Century: Formula and Beikost." *Journal of Nutrition* 131.2 (2001): 409s-20s. Print.

3. "Breastfeeding Report Card." *Centers for Disease Control and Prevention.* Centers for Disease Control and Prevention, 27 Jan. 2012. Web. 27 June 2012. <http://www.cdc.gov/breastfeeding/data/reportcard/reportcard2010.htm>.

4. Ibid.

5. Prentice, Ann. "Constituents of human milk." *Food and Nutrition Bulletin.* The United Nations University Press. 17.4 (1996). Print.

6. "Russian Woman Gets Three Years for Poisoning Son with Breast Milk." *RIA Novosti.* RIA Novosti, 30 Dec. 2011. Web. 27 June 2012. <http://en.rian.ru/crime/20111230/170562565.html>.

7. Fisher, Denise. "Social Drugs and Breastfeeding." *Health E-Learning.* N.p., n.d. Web. 27 June 2012. <http://www.health-e-learning.com/resources/articles/40-social-drugs-and-breastfeeding>.

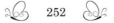

8. Allen, Peter. "French Vegan Couple Whose Baby Died of Vitamin Deficiency after Being Fed Solely on Breast Milk Face Jail for Child Neglect." *The Daily Mail*. N.p., 30 Mar. 2011. Web. 27 June 2012. <http://www.dailymail.co.uk/news/article-1371172/French-vegan-couple-face-jail-child-neglect-baby-died-vitamin-deficiency.html>.

9. Yildiz, Faiih. *Phytoestrogens in Functional Foods*. Boca Raton: CRC, 2006. Print.

10. Setchell, K. D. "Isoflavone Content of Infant Formulas and the Metabolic Fate of These Early Phytoestrogens in Early Life." *American Journal of Clinical Nutrition* 68.6 Supplemental (1998): 1453S-461S. Print.

11. Fallon, Sally. "Soy Infant Formula: Birth Control Pills for Babies." *Weston A Price Foundation*. N.p., 19 Oct. 2002. Web. 28 June 2012. <http://www.westonaprice.org/soy-alert/soy-formula-birth-control-pills-for-babies>.

12. "Hidden Sources of MSG." *Truth in Labeling*. Truth in Labeling Campaign, 01 Feb. 2011. Web. 28 June 2012. <http://www.truthinlabeling.org/hiddensources.html>.

13. Iannotti, Lora L., Robert E. Black, Maureen M. Black, and James M. Tielsch. "Iron Supplementation in Early Childhood: Health Benefits and Risks." *American Journal of Clinical Nutrition* 84.6 (2006): 1261-276. Print.

14. Oppenheimer, Stephen J. "Iron and Its Relation to Immunity and Infectious Disease." *Journal of Nutrition* 131.2 (2001): 616S-35S. Print.

Chapter 10: Baby's First Foods

1. Brodie, Michelle. "Cultural Aspects of Starting Solids." *New Beginnings* 18.2 (2001): 64-65. Print.

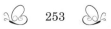

2. Small, Meredith F. *Our Babies, Ourselves: How Biology and Culture Shape the Way We Parent.* New York: Anchor, 1998. Print.

3. Allbriton, Jill. "The Smorgasbord Experiment." *Wise Traditions in Food, Farming and the Healing Arts* Winter (2009). Print.

4. Zoppi G, Andreotti F, Pajno-Ferrara F, Njai DM, Gaburro D. "Exocrine pancreas function in premature and full term neonates." *Pediatric Research.* 6 (1972):880-6.

5. Gillard BK, Simbala JA, Goodglick L. "Reference intervals for amylase isoenzymes in serum and plasma of infants and children." *Clinical Chemistry.* 29 (1983):119-23.

6. Tye, J. G., R. C. Karn, and A. D. Merritt. "Differential Expression of Salivary (Amy1) and Pancreatic (Amy2) Human Amylase Loci in Prenatal and Postnatal Development." *Journal of Medical Genetics* 13.2 (1976): 96-102. Print.

7. Otsuki, Makoto, Hosai Yuu, Susumu Saeki, and Shigeaki Baba. "The Characteristics of Amylase Activity and the Isoamylase Pattern in Serum and Urine of Infants and Children." *European Journal of Pediatrics* 125.3 (1977): 175-80. Print.

8. Campbell-McBride, Natasha. *Gut and Psychology Syndrome: Natural Treatment for Autism, Dyspraxia, A.D.D., Dyslexia, A.D.H.D., Depression, Schizophrenia.* Cambridge, U.K.: Medinform Pub., 2010. Print.

9. Fallon, Sally, and Mary Enig. "Feeding Babies." *Weston A Price Foundation.* Weston A Price Foundation, 31 Dec. 2001. Web. 28 June 2012. <http://www.westonaprice.org/childrens-health/feeding-babies>.

10. Ibid.

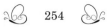

Photo Credit

Grain-FreeApple Pancake Rings: (c) Depositphotos.com/Monika Adamczyk

Barbeque Sauce: (c) Depositphotos.com/Stephanie Frey

Ceviche: (c) Depositphotos.com/Tono Balaguer

Chicken Liver Pate': (c) Depositphotos.com/Marco Mayer

Chinese Tomato and Eggs: (c) Depositphotos.com/Asimojet

Clam Chowder with Bacon and Green Chiles: (c) Depositphotos.com/Lynn
    Bendickson

Cranberry Relish: (c) Depositphotos.com/Elena Elisseeva

Crustless Crab Quiche: (c) Depositphotos.com/Nikolay Mikhalchenko

Dill Pickle Relish: (c) Depositphotos.com/Ольга Кригер

Egg Drop Soup: (c) Depositphotos.com/Denis Tabler

Egg and Roe Salad: (c) Depositphotos.com/Ольга Кригер

Eggs Poached in Marinara: (c) Depositphotos.com/Piccia Neri

Egg-Stravagant Breakfast Smoothie: (c) Depositphotos.com/Ivonne Wierink

Feta Egg Scramble: (c) Depositphotos.com/Barbara Helgason

Fizzy Lemonade: (c) Depositphotos.com/Olga Miltsova

Blender Hollandaise Sauce: (c) Depositphotos.com/Ildiko Papp

Homemade Almond Milk: (c) Depositphotos.com/WimL

Homemade Broth: (c) Depositphotos.com/Андрей Музыка

Sunshine Ketchup: (c) Depositphotos.com/Ольга Кригер

Liver & Onions: (c) Depositphotos.com/Svetlana Kolpakova

Make-Ahead Frozen Meatballs: (c) Depositphotos.com/Elena Elisseeva

Tantalizing Mayonnaise: (c) Depositphotos.com/Ольга Кригер

Parmesan Crisps: (c) Depositphotos.com/Monkey Business

Smoked Salmon Mousse: (c) Depositphotos.com/timolina

Scallops and Bacon: (c) Depositphotos.com/I Fong

Beef Tongue Taco Meat: (c) Depositphotos.com/Beth Swanson

Homemade Taco Seasoning: (c) Depositphotos.com/Mike Truchon

Tzatziki Sauce: (c) Depositphotos.com/Ingrid Heczko